HOW TO STRENGTHEN YOUR BONES AND MUSCLES

The Ultimate Bone and Muscle Strengthening Program for Osteoporosis Prevention and Management

Curtis Wood

Copyright © 2024 by Curtis Wood

Table of Content

Introduction

This book, "How to Strengthen Your Bones and Muscles: The Ultimate Bone and Muscle Strengthening Program for Osteoporosis Prevention and Management," is your guide to better bone and muscle health. If you're reading this, you're likely interested in taking proactive steps to improve your health, and that's a great place to start. Strong bones and muscles are essential for an active and healthy life, especially as we grow older. This book will help you understand, prevent, and manage osteoporosis while also teaching you how to build and maintain strong muscles.

Osteoporosis, often known as the "silent disease," weakens bones and makes them more likely to fracture. It affects millions of people around the world, particularly older adults and postmenopausal women. However, osteoporosis is not something you have to accept as inevitable. With the right knowledge and changes to your lifestyle, you can take control of your bone health and greatly reduce your risk of developing this condition.

In this book, you'll learn about the fascinating functions of bones and muscles. You will understand how your bones grow and repair themselves, and the crucial role muscles play in supporting them. We will cover the various factors that influence bone density and muscle strength, including genetics, age, diet, and physical activity. With this knowledge, you can make better choices for your health.

Nutrition is key to maintaining strong bones and muscles. We will guide you through the essential vitamins and minerals your body needs, such as calcium, vitamin D, and magnesium. You'll discover the best food sources for these nutrients and learn how to create a balanced diet that supports your bone and muscle health. Additionally, we'll discuss the importance of protein in preserving muscle mass and how to include it in your meals.

Exercise is another crucial element of bone and muscle health. This book introduces you to various exercises that help build and maintain bone density and muscle strength. From weight-bearing exercises and strength training to routines for flexibility and balance, you will find practical advice and step-by-step instructions to get you started. Whether you're new to exercise or have some experience, there's something here for you.

Beyond nutrition and exercise, we will discuss important lifestyle changes that can improve your bone and muscle health. You'll learn about the negative effects of smoking and excessive alcohol consumption, as well as the importance of managing stress. We will also provide tips on preventing falls and fractures, which are common concerns for people with osteoporosis.

Throughout this book, you'll find inspiring stories and case studies of individuals who have improved their bone and muscle health. Their experiences show that it's never too late to make positive changes. By following the advice and strategies in this book, you too can increase your bone density, strengthen your muscles, and enhance your overall well-being.

Lastly, we will talk about how to work effectively with healthcare providers to monitor your bone density and muscle mass and explore medication and alternative therapies for managing osteoporosis. Our aim is to give you the knowledge and tools you need to make informed decisions about your health and take proactive steps toward a stronger, healthier future.

Chapter 1: Understanding Osteoporosis

Osteoporosis is a condition that weakens bones, making them fragile and more likely to break. It's often called the "silent disease" because it develops slowly over time and usually doesn't have any symptoms until a bone breaks. This can be a fracture from a minor fall, or even from something as simple as a sneeze or a sudden movement. Understanding osteoporosis is the first step in preventing and managing it.

Bones are living tissues that are constantly being broken down and rebuilt. In our early years, our bodies make new bones faster than they break down old bones, so our bone mass increases. Most people reach their peak bone mass in their late 20s. After that, bone remodeling continues, but you lose slightly more bone mass than you gain. For some people, this bone loss happens too quickly or bone replacement occurs too slowly, leading to osteoporosis.

Osteoporosis affects millions of people worldwide. While it can affect anyone, it is most common in older women, particularly after menopause. This is because the hormone estrogen, which helps protect bones, decreases sharply when women reach menopause. Men also can develop osteoporosis, but it usually occurs later in life and progresses more slowly.

Several factors can increase your risk of developing osteoporosis. Age is a significant factor, as the risk increases as you get older. Gender is another factor, with women being more prone to osteoporosis than men. Family history also plays a role; if your parents or grandparents had osteoporosis or hip fractures, your risk is higher. Other risk factors include low body weight, certain medical conditions (like rheumatoid arthritis), and certain medications (such as long-term use of steroids).

Lifestyle choices can also impact your bone health. Smoking and excessive alcohol consumption can increase your risk of osteoporosis. A diet low in calcium and vitamin D, which are crucial for bone health, can also contribute to the disease. Lack of physical activity is another risk factor, as regular exercise helps to strengthen bones and muscles.

Diagnosing osteoporosis typically involves a bone density test, which measures the density of bones in various parts of the body, such as the hip and spine. This test is quick and painless, and it can help doctors determine whether you have osteoporosis or are at risk of developing it. Early detection is essential because it allows for timely intervention to prevent fractures and further bone loss.

Preventing osteoporosis involves several strategies. A diet rich in calcium and vitamin D is vital. Calcium helps build and maintain strong bones, while vitamin D improves calcium absorption in the body. Dairy products, leafy green vegetables, and fortified foods are excellent sources of calcium. Sunlight is a natural source of vitamin D, but it can also be found in fatty fish, liver, and fortified foods. Regular exercise is also crucial for bone health. Weight-bearing exercises, like walking, jogging, and dancing, help build and maintain bone density. Strength training exercises, such as lifting weights, can also help by increasing muscle mass and strength, which supports and protects bones. Balance and flexibility exercises, like tai chi and yoga, can help prevent falls by improving stability and coordination.

In addition to diet and exercise, lifestyle changes can help reduce the risk of osteoporosis. Avoiding smoking and limiting alcohol intake are important steps. Smoking can decrease bone mass, and excessive alcohol can interfere with the balance of calcium in the body. Managing stress through relaxation techniques, such as meditation or deep-breathing exercises, can also have a positive effect on your overall health, including your bones.

For those already diagnosed with osteoporosis, treatment options are available to help manage the condition and prevent fractures. Medications can help slow bone loss and increase bone density. Working with your healthcare provider to develop a personalized plan is crucial. This plan may include medication, dietary supplements, and a specific exercise program tailored to your needs.

Understanding osteoporosis is crucial for taking control of your bone health. By learning about the factors that contribute to this condition and adopting a proactive approach, you can significantly reduce your risk and lead a healthier, more active life. Whether you are looking to prevent osteoporosis or manage it effectively, the information in this book will equip you with the knowledge and tools you need to make informed decisions about your health.

Chapter 2: The Importance of Bone and Muscle Health

Bone and muscle health are vital to our overall well-being. Strong bones and muscles allow us to move freely and perform everyday tasks with ease. They provide the support and stability our bodies need to stay active and healthy. Understanding the importance of maintaining strong bones and muscles can help us lead longer, more vibrant lives. Bones form the structure of our bodies. They protect our internal organs, like the brain, heart, and lungs. Bones also store essential minerals, such as calcium and phosphorus, which are released into the body when needed. Without strong bones, our bodies would be weak and fragile, making us more susceptible to injuries and diseases.

Muscles are equally important. They are attached to bones and work with them to allow movement. Muscles also help maintain our posture and balance. Strong muscles support our bones and joints, reducing the risk of injuries. They also help with blood circulation and maintaining a healthy weight by burning calories even when we're at rest.

As we age, our bones and muscles naturally lose strength. This process can start as early as our 30s. Without proper care, this weakening can lead to conditions like osteoporosis and sarcopenia, which is the loss of muscle mass. These conditions can severely impact our quality of life, making simple activities like walking, lifting objects, or even standing up difficult and painful.

Maintaining strong bones and muscles is crucial for preventing these conditions. A healthy diet and regular exercise are key components of this maintenance. Eating foods rich in calcium and vitamin D helps keep bones strong. Calcium is found in dairy products, leafy greens, and fortified foods, while vitamin D is obtained from sunlight and certain foods like fatty fish and fortified milk.

Protein is essential for muscle health. It helps repair and build muscle tissues. Good sources of protein include meat, fish, eggs, beans, and nuts. Including protein in every meal can help maintain muscle mass, especially as we get older.

Exercise plays a vital role in maintaining bone and muscle health. Weight-bearing exercises, such as walking, running, and dancing, help build bone density. Strength training exercises, like lifting weights or using resistance bands, are excellent for building and maintaining muscle mass. These activities also improve balance and coordination, reducing the risk of falls and fractures.

Even if you haven't been active before, it's never too late to start. Begin with simple exercises and gradually increase the intensity and duration as you become more comfortable. Regular physical activity not only strengthens bones and muscles but also boosts energy levels, improves mood, and enhances overall health.

In addition to diet and exercise, lifestyle choices can significantly impact bone and muscle health. Smoking and excessive alcohol consumption can weaken bones and muscles, so avoiding these habits is crucial. Managing stress through relaxation techniques, such as meditation and deep breathing, can also have a positive effect on your overall health.

Regular check-ups with your healthcare provider are important for monitoring bone and muscle health. Bone density tests can detect early signs of osteoporosis, allowing for timely intervention. Your doctor can also recommend supplements or medications if necessary to help maintain bone density and muscle mass.

For those already experiencing bone or muscle loss, it's essential to follow a personalized plan that may include dietary changes, exercise routines, and possibly medications. Working closely with your healthcare provider can help manage these conditions effectively and improve your quality of life.

Understanding the importance of bone and muscle health is the first step in taking control of your well-being. By making informed choices about your diet, exercise, and lifestyle, you can maintain strong bones and muscles throughout your life. This book provides you with the k

knowledge and tools needed to achieve this goal.

Chapter 3: The Science of Bone Strength

Bone strength is fundamental to our health and ability to move. Understanding how bones work can help us take better care of them. This section will explore the science behind bone strength, explaining how bones are formed, maintained, and why they sometimes weaken.

Bones are made of living tissue. They are constantly growing and changing. This process is known as remodeling, and it involves two types of cells: osteoblasts and osteoclasts. Osteoblasts are responsible for building new bone tissue, while osteoclasts break down old bone tissue. This continuous cycle of bone formation and resorption ensures that our bones stay strong and healthy.

During childhood and adolescence, the body makes new bone faster than it breaks down old bone, leading to an increase in bone mass. Most people reach their peak bone mass around their late 20s. After this point, the balance between bone formation and bone breakdown shifts, and bone mass gradually begins to decline.

Several factors influence bone strength. Genetics plays a significant role in determining peak bone mass. If your parents had strong bones, you are more likely to have strong bones as well. Gender is another factor; women generally have lower peak bone mass than men and are more likely to develop osteoporosis later in life. This is partly due to hormonal differences, especially the drop in estrogen levels during menopause, which accelerates bone loss.

Nutrition is crucial for bone health. Calcium and vitamin D are two essential nutrients for maintaining strong bones. Calcium is a primary building block of bone tissue, while vitamin D helps the body absorb calcium. Without enough calcium and vitamin D, bones can become weak and brittle. Other nutrients, such as magnesium, phosphorus, and vitamin K, also play vital roles in bone health.

Physical activity is another key factor in maintaining bone strength. Weight-bearing exercises, such as walking, running, and lifting weights, stimulate bone formation and help maintain bone density. When muscles pull on bones during physical activity, it signals the body to produce more bone tissue, making bones stronger. This is why regular exercise is so important for bone health, especially as we age.

Hormones also play a significant role in bone health. Estrogen and testosterone are hormones that help maintain bone density. When levels of these hormones decrease, as they do during menopause in women and with aging in men, bone loss can accelerate. Thyroid hormones and parathyroid hormones also affect bone metabolism.

An imbalance in these hormones can lead to bone loss and increase the risk of osteoporosis.

Bone diseases, such as osteoporosis, occur when the balance between bone formation and bone breakdown is disrupted. In osteoporosis, bones become porous and fragile, making them more prone to fractures. This condition often develops without any symptoms until a bone breaks, which is why it's called the "silent disease." Understanding the science behind bone strength can help us take preventive measures to protect our bones and maintain their health.

Preventing bone loss involves several strategies. Ensuring an adequate intake of calcium and vitamin D through diet and supplements is essential. Foods rich in calcium include dairy products, leafy green vegetables, nuts, and seeds. Vitamin D can be obtained from sunlight exposure, fatty fish, and fortified foods. In some cases, supplements may be necessary to meet daily requirements.

Regular physical activity is crucial for maintaining bone strength. Weight-bearing and resistance exercises are particularly effective in stimulating bone formation. Activities such as walking, jogging, dancing, and weight lifting help keep bones dense and strong. Balance and flexibility exercises, like yoga and tai chi, can help prevent falls, which are a common cause of fractures in people with weak bones.

Avoiding smoking and limiting alcohol consumption is also important for bone health. Smoking can reduce bone mass, while excessive alcohol can interfere with the body's ability to absorb calcium. Managing stress and getting enough sleep are also important, as chronic stress and lack of sleep can negatively impact bone health. Regular check-ups with your healthcare provider can help monitor bone density and detect any early signs of bone loss. Bone density tests, such as DEXA scans, measure the density of bones in the hip and spine and can help identify osteoporosis before fractures occur. If you are at risk of osteoporosis, your doctor may recommend medications to help maintain bone density and reduce the risk of fractures.

Understanding the science of bone strength empowers us to take proactive steps to protect our bones. By focusing on a balanced diet, regular exercise, and healthy lifestyle choices, we can maintain strong bones and reduce the risk of osteoporosis. This knowledge, combined with the strategies outlined in this book, will help you build a solid foundation for lifelong bone health.

Chapter 4: Factors Affecting Bone and Muscle Health

Bone and muscle health are critical for our overall well-being. They enable us to move, support our body, and protect our organs. Many factors can influence the health of our bones and muscles, and understanding these can help us make better choices to keep them strong. Let's explore these factors in detail.

1. Age

As we age, our bones and muscles naturally lose strength. This process starts in our 30s and accelerates as we get older. For bones, this happens because the balance between bone formation and bone breakdown shifts, leading to a gradual loss of bone density, for muscles, aging leads to a loss of muscle mass and strength, a condition known as sarcopenia. This is why older adults are more prone to fractures and muscle weakness.

2. Genetics

Genetics plays a significant role in determining bone density and muscle strength. If your parents or grandparents had strong bones and muscles, you are more likely to have them too. Conversely, a family history of osteoporosis or weak muscles can increase your risk of these conditions. While we can't change our genetics, being aware of our family history can help us take preventive measures.

3. Gender

Women are generally more susceptible to bone loss than men, especially after menopause. This is because estrogen, a hormone that helps protect bones, decreases significantly during menopause, leading to faster bone loss. Men also experience bone loss with age, but usually at a slower rate. Both men and women can benefit from taking steps to maintain bone and muscle health throughout their lives.

4. Nutrition

A balanced diet is essential for maintaining strong bones and muscles. Calcium and vitamin D are particularly important for bone health. Calcium is a primary building block of bone tissue, while vitamin D helps the body absorb calcium. Dairy products, leafy green vegetables, and fortified foods are excellent sources of calcium. Sunlight, fatty fish, and fortified foods provide vitamin D. For muscle health, protein is crucial. It helps build and repair muscle tissues. Good sources of protein include meat, fish, eggs, beans, and nuts.

5. Physical Activity

Regular exercise is one of the best ways to maintain bone and muscle health. Weight-bearing exercises, such as walking, running, and dancing, help build and maintain bone density. Strength training exercises, like lifting weights or using resistance bands, are excellent for building and maintaining muscle mass. These activities also improve balance and coordination, which can prevent falls and fractures.

6. Hormones

Hormones play a vital role in bone and muscle health. Estrogen and testosterone help maintain bone density. When the levels of these hormones decrease, bone loss can accelerate. Thyroid hormones and parathyroid hormones also affect bone metabolism. An imbalance in these hormones can lead to bone loss and an increased risk of osteoporosis. Similarly, hormones like growth hormone and insulin-like growth factor are important for muscle growth and maintenance.

7. Lifestyle Choices

Certain lifestyle choices can impact bone and muscle health. Smoking is harmful to bones because it reduces blood flow to the bones and decreases the body's ability to absorb calcium. Excessive alcohol consumption can also weaken bones and muscles by interfering with the balance of calcium and other nutrients in the body. Maintaining a healthy weight is important as well. Being underweight can increase the risk of bone loss while being overweight can put extra strain on bones and muscles.

8. Medical Conditions and Medications

Certain medical conditions, such as rheumatoid arthritis and chronic kidney disease, can affect bone and muscle health. Some medications, like long-term use of corticosteroids, can also lead to bone loss and muscle weakness. It's important to discuss with your healthcare provider how your medical conditions and medications might affect your bones and muscles and what steps you can take to mitigate any negative effects.

9. Falls and Injuries

Falls and injuries can have a significant impact on bone and muscle health, especially in older adults. A fall can lead to fractures, which can be debilitating. Strengthening muscles and improving balance through regular exercise can help prevent falls. Using assistive devices, such as handrails and non-slip mats, can also reduce the risk of falls at home.

10. Stress and Sleep

Chronic stress can negatively impact bone and muscle health. High levels of the stress hormone cortisol can lead to bone loss and muscle weakness.

Getting enough sleep is also crucial, as sleep is the time when the body repairs and builds tissues, including bones and muscles. Aim for 7-9 hours of quality sleep each night to support your overall health.

Many factors affect bone and muscle health, from age and genetics to lifestyle choices and medical conditions. By understanding these factors, we can take proactive steps to maintain strong bones and muscles. This includes eating a balanced diet rich in calcium, vitamin D, and protein, engaging in regular physical activity, avoiding smoking and excessive alcohol consumption, and managing stress and sleep. Regular check-ups with your healthcare provider can also help monitor bone and muscle health and catch any issues early. By taking these steps, we can ensure that our bones and muscles remain strong, allowing us to lead active, healthy lives for years to come.

Chapter 5: Nutritional Strategies for Strong Bones

Eating the right foods is crucial for maintaining strong bones. Our bones need a variety of nutrients to stay healthy and strong. This section will explain which nutrients are important for bone health, what foods are rich in these nutrients, and how to incorporate them into your diet.

Calcium: The Building Block of Bones

Calcium is the most important mineral for bone health. It makes up a large part of our bones and helps keep them strong. Most adults need about 1,000 milligrams of calcium per day, and this amount increases to 1,200 milligrams per day for women over 50 and men over 70.

Good sources of calcium include:

- Dairy products like milk, cheese, and yogurt

- Leafy green vegetables like kale, broccoli, and spinach

- Fortified foods such as orange juice, cereals, and plant-based milks

- Almonds and sesame seeds

- Fish with edible bones, like sardines and canned salmon

Vitamin D: Helping the Body Absorb Calcium

Vitamin D helps our bodies absorb calcium. Without enough vitamin D, even if you consume a lot of calcium, your body can't use it effectively. Adults need about 600 to 800 international units (IU) of vitamin D per day.

Sources of vitamin D include:

- Sunlight: Our skin makes vitamin D when exposed to sunlight. Spending about 10-30 minutes in the sun several times a week can help, but the amount needed can vary based on skin tone, location, and time of year.
- Fatty fish like salmon, mackerel, and tuna
- Fortified foods such as milk, orange juice, and cereals
- Egg yolks
- Supplements, if needed, after consulting with a healthcare provider

Protein: Building and Repairing Bone and Muscle

Protein is essential for the growth, repair, and maintenance of bone and muscle tissues. Adults should aim for about 0.8 grams of protein per kilogram of body weight each day.

Good sources of protein include:
- Lean meats like chicken, turkey, and beef

- Fish and seafood
- Eggs
- Dairy products such as milk, cheese, and yogurt
- Plant-based sources like beans, lentils, tofu, nuts, and seeds

Magnesium: Supporting Bone Structure

Magnesium helps with bone formation and plays a role in converting vitamin D into its active form, which aids calcium absorption. Adults need about 310-420 milligrams of magnesium per day.

Sources of magnesium include:
- Nuts and seeds, especially almonds, pumpkin seeds, and sunflower seeds
- Whole grains like brown rice, quinoa, and whole wheat
- Leafy green vegetables such as spinach and Swiss chard
- Legumes like black beans, lentils, and chickpeas

- Fish, particularly mackerel and salmon

Phosphorus: Partnering with Calcium

Phosphorus works with calcium to build strong bones and teeth. Adults need about 700 milligrams of phosphorus per day.

Sources of phosphorus include:
- Meat and poultry
- Fish and seafood
- Dairy products
- Nuts and seeds
- Whole grains

Vitamin K: Helping Bone Mineralization

Vitamin K is important for bone mineralization, the process that helps form strong bones. Adults need about 90-120 micrograms of vitamin K per day.

Sources of vitamin K include:
- Leafy green vegetables like kale, spinach, and broccoli
- Brussels sprouts
- Green beans
- Soybeans and soybean oil
- Eggs

Incorporating Bone-Healthy Foods into Your Diet
To ensure you get enough of these essential nutrients, consider these tips for incorporating bone-healthy foods into your diet:

1. Balanced Meals: Aim to include a source of calcium, vitamin D, and protein in every meal. For example, have a spinach and cheese omelet for breakfast, a salmon salad for lunch, and grilled chicken with broccoli and quinoa for dinner.

2. Snacking Smart: Choose snacks that are rich in bone-building nutrients. Yogurt with nuts, cheese with whole-grain crackers, or a handful of almonds can provide a boost of calcium, protein, and magnesium.

3. Fortified Foods: Include fortified foods in your diet, such as calcium-fortified orange juice, cereals, and plant-based milk. These can help fill any gaps in your nutrient intake.

4. Variety of Sources: Try to get your nutrients from a variety of sources. Different foods provide different nutrients, and a varied diet ensures you're getting a broad spectrum of vitamins and minerals.

5. Cooking Techniques: Use cooking methods that retain nutrients, such as steaming vegetables instead of boiling them, which can cause some nutrients to leach out into the water.

6. Supplements: If you have difficulty getting enough of certain nutrients from food alone, talk to your healthcare provider about supplements. This is especially important for vitamin D, which can be hard to get from food and sunlight alone, especially in certain climates or seasons.

Strong bones require a mix of essential nutrients, including calcium, vitamin D, protein, magnesium, phosphorus, and vitamin K. By eating a balanced diet rich in these nutrients and making thoughtful food choices, you can support your bone health and reduce the risk of osteoporosis and fractures. Incorporate a variety of nutrient-dense foods into your daily meals and snacks, and consider fortified foods and supplements if necessary. With these nutritional strategies, you can help ensure your bones stay strong and healthy throughout your life.

Chapter 6: Essential Vitamins and Minerals

Vitamins and minerals are vital for our bodies. They help us grow, stay healthy, and have enough energy. Each vitamin and mineral has a specific job, and together they keep our bodies working well. Let's explore some of the most important vitamins and minerals, what they do, and where to find them.

1. Vitamin A

Vitamin A is essential for good vision, a strong immune system, and healthy skin. It helps our eyes adjust to light changes and keeps them moist.

Sources of vitamin A include:

- Carrots

- Sweet potatoes
- Spinach
- Kale
- Liver
- Fish

2. Vitamin B

The B vitamins are a group of eight different vitamins that help our bodies convert food into energy. They also support brain function and cell metabolism. The main B vitamins are B1 (thiamine), B2 (riboflavin), B3 (niacin), B5 (pantothenic acid), B6 (pyridoxine), B7 (biotin), B9 (folate), and B12 (cobalamin).

Sources of B vitamins include:
- Whole grains
- Meat and poultry
- Fish
- Eggs
- Dairy products

- Leafy green vegetables
- Beans and peas
- Nuts and seeds

3. Vitamin C

Vitamin C is important for the growth and repair of tissues. It helps heal wounds, strengthens the immune system, and acts as an antioxidant, protecting cells from damage.

Sources of vitamin C include:
- Oranges
- Strawberries
- Kiwi
- Bell peppers
- Broccoli
- Brussels sprouts
- Tomatoes

4. Vitamin D

Vitamin D helps our bodies absorb calcium, which is necessary for strong bones and teeth. It also supports the immune system and helps reduce inflammation.

Sources of vitamin D include:
- Sunlight (our bodies produce vitamin D when exposed to sunlight)
- Fatty fish like salmon and mackerel
- Fortified foods such as milk, orange juice, and cereals
- Egg yolks
- Supplements, if needed

5. Vitamin E

Vitamin E acts as an antioxidant, protecting cells from damage. It also supports the immune system and helps keep skin and eyes healthy.

Sources of vitamin E include:

- Nuts and seeds, especially almonds and sunflower seeds
- Spinach
- Broccoli
- Vegetable oils like sunflower, safflower, and wheat germ oil
- Fortified cereals

6. Vitamin K

Vitamin K is crucial for blood clotting, which helps wounds heal properly. It also plays a role in bone health.

Sources of vitamin K include:
- Leafy green vegetables like kale, spinach, and broccoli
- Brussels sprouts
- Green beans
- Soybeans and soybean oil
- Eggs

7. Calcium

Calcium is essential for strong bones and teeth. It also helps with muscle function, nerve signaling, and blood clotting.

Sources of calcium include:
- Dairy products like milk, cheese, and yogurt
- Leafy green vegetables such as kale and broccoli
- Fortified foods like orange juice, cereals, and plant-based milks
- Almonds
- Sardines and canned salmon (with bones)

8. Iron

Iron is important for making hemoglobin, a protein in red blood cells that carries oxygen throughout the body. It also supports muscle metabolism and healthy connective tissue.

Sources of iron include:
- Red meat

- Poultry
- Fish and seafood
- Beans and lentils
- Spinach
- Fortified cereals
- Tofu

9. Magnesium

Magnesium is involved in over 300 biochemical reactions in the body. It supports muscle and nerve function, regulates blood sugar levels, and helps maintain strong bones.

Sources of magnesium include:
- Nuts and seeds, especially almonds and pumpkin seeds
- Whole grains like brown rice, quinoa, and whole wheat
- Leafy green vegetables such as spinach and Swiss chard
- Legumes like black beans and chickpeas

- Fish, particularly mackerel and salmon

10. Potassium

Potassium helps regulate fluid balance, muscle contractions, and nerve signals. It can also help reduce blood pressure and protect against stroke.

Sources of potassium include:
- Bananas
- Oranges and orange juice
- Potatoes
- Spinach
- Tomatoes
- Beans and lentils
- Yogurt

11. Zinc

Zinc is crucial for the immune system, wound healing, DNA synthesis, and cell division. It also supports normal growth and development during pregnancy, childhood, and adolescence.

Sources of zinc include:
- Meat and poultry
- Seafood, especially oysters
- Beans and lentils
- Nuts and seeds
- Dairy products
- Whole grains

12. Selenium

Selenium acts as an antioxidant, helping protect cells from damage. It also plays a role in metabolism and thyroid function.

Sources of selenium include:
- Brazil nuts
- Seafood, especially tuna and shrimp
- Meat and poultry
- Eggs
- Dairy products
- Whole grains

Incorporating Vitamins and Minerals into Your Diet

To ensure you get enough essential vitamins and minerals, aim for a balanced and varied diet. Here are some tips to help you incorporate these nutrients into your meals:

1. Eat a Rainbow: Include a variety of colorful fruits and vegetables in your diet. Different colors often indicate different nutrients, so a colorful plate can help ensure you're getting a broad range of vitamins and minerals.

2. Choose Whole Foods: Opt for whole grains, lean proteins, and fresh produce over processed foods. Whole foods are generally more nutrient-dense and less likely to contain added sugars and unhealthy fats.

3. Cook at Home: Preparing meals at home allows you to control the ingredients and cooking methods, helping you create healthier, nutrient-rich meals.

4. Snack Wisely: Choose nutrient-dense snacks like yogurt with fruit, a handful of nuts, or carrot sticks with hummus to boost your intake of essential vitamins and minerals.

5. Read Labels: When buying packaged foods, read the labels to check for added vitamins and minerals. Fortified foods can help fill nutrient gaps in your diet.

6. Stay Hydrated: Drink plenty of water and include hydrating foods like fruits and vegetables to support overall health and help your body absorb nutrients more effectively.

Essential vitamins and minerals are the building blocks of a healthy body. They support everything from strong bones and muscles to good vision and a robust immune system. By eating a balanced and varied diet rich in fruits, vegetables, whole grains, lean proteins, and healthy fats, you can ensure you get the nutrients your body needs to thrive. Remember, a colorful plate is a healthy plate, and small changes in your diet can make a big difference in your overall well-being.

Chapter 7: The Role of Protein in Muscle Maintenance

Protein is one of the most important nutrients our bodies need, especially for maintaining strong and healthy muscles. Understanding how protein works and why it's so crucial can help us make better food choices and keep our muscles in top shape.

What is Protein?

Protein is made up of building blocks called amino acids. There are 20 different amino acids, and our bodies need all of them to function properly. Nine of these amino acids are essential, meaning we must get them from our diet because our bodies can't make them on their own.

How Does Protein Help Muscles?

Muscles are made of protein. When we eat protein, our bodies break it down into amino acids, which are then used to build and repair muscle tissues. This process is continuous; our muscles are always being broken down and rebuilt. Eating enough protein ensures that our bodies have the necessary building blocks to maintain and repair muscles.

Why is Protein Important for Muscle Maintenance?

1. Muscle Repair and Growth: After exercise or any physical activity, our muscles need to repair themselves. Protein provides the amino acids required for this repair process, helping muscles recover and grow stronger.

2. Preventing Muscle Loss: As we age, we naturally lose muscle mass. This process, called sarcopenia, can be slowed down by eating enough protein.

Ensuring an adequate protein intake helps maintain muscle mass and strength, reducing the risk of frailty and falls in older adults.

3. Energy Source: While carbohydrates and fats are the body's main sources of energy, protein can also be used for energy if needed. This is especially important during long periods of physical activity or when the body is under stress.

4. Satiety and Weight Management: Protein-rich foods help us feel full longer. This can be beneficial for weight management, as it helps control appetite and reduce overall calorie intake.

How Much Protein Do We Need?

The amount of protein we need can vary based on age, sex, physical activity level, and overall health. However, a general guideline is to consume 0.8 grams of protein per kilogram of body weight per day. For those who are very active or looking to build muscle, the requirement may be higher, around 1.2 to 2.0 grams per kilogram of body weight.

Sources of Protein

There are many sources of protein, both animal-based and plant-based. Including a variety of these in your diet can help ensure you get all the essential amino acids.

Animal-Based Sources

- Lean meats such as chicken, turkey, and beef
- Fish and seafood
- Eggs
- Dairy products like milk, cheese, and yogurt

Plant-Based Sources

- Beans and legumes such as lentils, chickpeas, and black beans
- Tofu and tempeh

- Nuts and seeds like almonds, walnuts, chia seeds, and sunflower seeds
- Whole grains such as quinoa, brown rice, and oats

Incorporating Protein into Your Diet

Adding protein to your diet doesn't have to be complicated. Here are some simple ways to make sure you're getting enough:

1. Balanced Meals: Include a source of protein in every meal. For breakfast, try eggs or Greek yogurt with nuts. For lunch and dinner, add chicken, fish, or beans to your salads, soups, or stir-fries.

2. Protein-Rich Snacks: Choose snacks that are high in protein. Some great options are cheese sticks, a handful of nuts, a protein shake, or hummus with veggie sticks.

3. Mix It Up: Don't rely on just one source of protein. Eat a variety of protein-rich foods to ensure you're getting a good mix of amino acids and other nutrients.

4. Plan Ahead: Preparing meals and snacks in advance can help you make sure you always have protein-rich options available. Cook extra portions of chicken or fish to use in salads or sandwiches throughout the week, or batch-cook a big pot of lentil soup.

5. Read Labels: When buying packaged foods, check the labels for protein content. Some foods are fortified with extra protein, which can help you meet your daily needs.

Special Considerations

- Vegetarians and Vegans: Plant-based eaters can get enough protein by combining different sources. For example, eating beans with rice or hummus with whole-grain bread ensures you're getting a complete set of amino acids.

- Athletes and Active Individuals: If you're very active or trying to build muscle, you may need more protein. Spread your protein intake throughout the day and consider adding a protein shake after workouts to support muscle recovery.

- Older Adults: As we age, our bodies become less efficient at using protein. Older adults should aim for a slightly higher protein intake to help maintain muscle mass and strength.

Protein is essential for maintaining strong and healthy muscles. It helps repair and build muscle tissues, prevents muscle loss, and provides energy. Including a variety of protein-rich foods in your diet ensures you get all the essential amino acids your body needs. Whether you're young or old, active or sedentary, making sure you eat enough protein is a key part of staying healthy and strong.

Chapter 8: Exercise and Bone Health

Exercise is essential for keeping our bones strong and healthy. Just like muscles, bones need to be worked and challenged to stay in good shape. Regular physical activity can help prevent bone loss, reduce the risk of fractures, and even improve our balance and coordination, which can prevent falls. Let's explore how exercise benefits our bones, what types of exercises are best, and how to get started with a bone-healthy fitness routine.

Why Exercise is Important for Bones

1. Building Bone Density: When we're young, exercise helps us build strong bones. Weight-bearing activities, like running and jumping,

stimulate bone growth and increase bone density. This is especially important during childhood and adolescence when bones are growing the fastest.

2. Preventing Bone Loss: As we age, our bones naturally lose density. Regular exercise can slow this process, helping to maintain bone strength and reduce the risk of osteoporosis, a condition where bones become weak and brittle.

3. Improving Balance and Coordination: Exercise not only strengthens bones but also improves muscle strength, balance, and coordination. This is crucial for preventing falls, which can lead to fractures, especially in older adults.

4. Enhancing Overall Health: Physical activity has many benefits beyond bone health. It improves cardiovascular health, boosts mood, helps control weight, and increases overall energy levels. When we feel good and have more energy, we're more

likely to stay active, creating a positive cycle of health and wellness.

Best Types of Exercises for Bone Health

1. Weight-Bearing Exercises: These are activities that make you move against gravity while staying upright. They help build and maintain bone density. Examples include:
   - Walking
   - Running or jogging
   - Hiking
   - Dancing
   - Jumping rope
   - Stair climbing

2. Strength Training: Also known as resistance training, this involves lifting weights or using resistance bands. Strength training not only builds muscle but also strengthens bones by putting stress

on them, which stimulates bone growth. Examples include:
  - Lifting free weights
  - Using weight machines
  - Bodyweight exercises like push-ups and squats
  - Resistance band exercises

3. Balance and Flexibility Exercises: These exercises improve coordination and flexibility, which helps prevent falls. They also keep joints healthy and muscles strong. Examples include:
  - Tai Chi
  - Yoga
  - Pilates
  - Balance drills like standing on one leg

4. High-Impact Activities: These exercises are particularly effective for building bone density. However, they may not be suitable for everyone, especially those with existing bone or joint issues. Examples include:

- Running or jogging
- High-impact aerobics
- Sports like basketball, tennis, and soccer

Getting Started with a Bone-Healthy Exercise Routine

1. Consult Your Doctor: Before starting any new exercise routine, especially if you have any health concerns or conditions, it's important to talk to your doctor. They can help you determine which exercises are safe and beneficial for you.

2. Start Slow: If you're new to exercise or haven't been active for a while, start slow and gradually increase the intensity and duration of your workouts. Begin with short walks or light strength training and build up over time.

3. Mix It Up: Incorporate a variety of exercises into your routine to keep it interesting and work different parts of your body. Combine weight-

bearing, strength training, and balance exercises for the best results.

4. Set Realistic Goals: Set achievable goals to stay motivated. Start with small, manageable targets, like walking for 20 minutes three times a week, and gradually increase as you become more comfortable and fit.

5. Listen to Your Body: Pay attention to how your body feels during and after exercise. It's normal to feel some soreness when you start a new exercise routine, but sharp pain or discomfort could be a sign that you're overdoing it or performing an exercise incorrectly. If something doesn't feel right, stop and seek advice from a fitness professional or healthcare provider.

6. Stay Consistent: Consistency is key to reaping the benefits of exercise. Make physical activity a regular part of your routine. Aim for at least 30

minutes of moderate-intensity exercise most days of the week. Even short, 10-minute bouts of activity can add up and make a difference.

Fun Ways to Stay Active

Exercise doesn't have to be a chore. Find activities you enjoy to make staying active fun and engaging. Here are some ideas:

- Join a Group: Participating in group fitness classes, walking clubs, or sports teams can make exercise more enjoyable and provide social support.
- Try New Activities: Explore different types of physical activities to find what you like best. Whether it's dancing, swimming, or hiking, trying new things can keep your routine fresh and exciting.
- Use Technology: Fitness apps and wearable devices can help you track your progress, set goals, and stay motivated. Many apps also offer guided workouts and fitness challenges.

- Make It a Habit: Incorporate physical activity into your daily routine. Take the stairs instead of the elevator, walk or bike to nearby destinations, or do simple exercises during TV commercials.

Exercise is crucial for maintaining strong, healthy bones throughout our lives. By engaging in weight-bearing, strength training, and balance exercises, we can build bone density, prevent bone loss, and improve our overall health and well-being. Starting an exercise routine may seem daunting, but by consulting with your doctor, starting slowly, and finding activities you enjoy, you can make physical activity a regular and enjoyable part of your life.

Chapter 9: Strength Training Techniques

Strength training, also known as resistance training or weight lifting, is an essential part of a healthy lifestyle. It helps build muscle, strengthens bones, and improves overall fitness. Whether you're a beginner or have some experience, understanding the right techniques can make your workouts more effective and safe. Let's explore different strength training techniques, how to do them properly, and the benefits they offer.

Why Strength Training is Important

1. Builds Muscle Mass: Strength training increases muscle size and strength. This not only makes you

stronger but also helps with daily activities, like carrying groceries or climbing stairs.

2. Strengthens Bones: Lifting weights puts stress on your bones, which helps them grow stronger and denser. This is crucial for preventing osteoporosis and reducing the risk of fractures.

3. Boosts Metabolism: Muscle tissue burns more calories than fat tissue, even when you're at rest. Strength training can increase your muscle mass, which in turn boosts your metabolism and helps with weight management.

4. Improves Mental Health: Exercise, including strength training, releases endorphins, which are chemicals in the brain that make you feel good. It can reduce stress, improve mood, and boost self-esteem.

Basic Strength Training Techniques

1. Bodyweight Exercises: These exercises use your body weight as resistance. They're great for beginners and can be done anywhere, without any equipment.

- Push-Ups: Start in a plank position with your hands shoulder-width apart. Lower your body until your chest almost touches the floor, then push back up. Keep your body in a straight line throughout the movement.

- Squats: Stand with your feet shoulder-width apart. Lower your body as if you're sitting back into a chair, keeping your chest up and your knees behind your toes. Return to the starting position.

- Lunges: Stand with your feet together. Step forward with one leg and lower your body until both knees are bent at a 90-degree angle. Push back up to the starting position and repeat with the other leg.

2. Free Weights: Using free weights like dumbbells and barbells allows for a wide range of motion and engages multiple muscles at once.

- Bicep Curls: Stand with a dumbbell in each hand, arms at your sides. Curl the weights up toward your shoulders, keeping your elbows close to your body. Lower the weights back down slowly.

- Shoulder Press: Hold a dumbbell in each hand at shoulder height with your palms facing forward. Press the weights overhead until your arms are fully extended, then lower them back to shoulder height.

- Deadlifts: Stand with your feet hip-width apart, holding a barbell in front of you. Bend at your hips and knees, keeping your back straight, and lower the barbell to the ground. Lift the barbell by straightening your hips and knees.

3. Weight Machines: These machines provide support and guide your movements, making them a good option for beginners or those recovering from injuries.

- Leg Press: Sit on the machine with your feet on the platform. Push the platform away by extending your legs, then slowly return to the starting position.

- Chest Press: Sit on the machine with the handles at chest height. Push the handles away from your chest until your arms are fully extended, then return to the starting position.

- Lat Pulldown: Sit at the machine with your knees secured under the pad. Grab the bar with a wide grip and pull it down toward your chest, then slowly let it return to the starting position.

4. Resistance Bands: These elastic bands provide resistance when stretched, offering a portable and versatile strength training option.

- Band Rows: Attach a resistance band to a sturdy object at chest height. Hold the band handles with both hands, step back to create tension, and pull the handles toward your chest, squeezing your shoulder blades together.

- Band Squats: Stand on the band with your feet shoulder-width apart, holding the handles at shoulder height. Perform a squat while keeping tension in the band.

- Band Push-Ups: Place the band across your back and hold the ends in your hands. Perform push-ups, keeping tension in the band to increase resistance.

Tips for Safe and Effective Strength Training

1. Warm Up: Always start with a warm-up to prepare your muscles and joints for exercise. A few minutes of light cardio, like walking or jogging, followed by dynamic stretches, can help prevent injuries.

2. Proper Form: Using the correct form is crucial to avoid injuries and get the most out of your workouts. If you're unsure about your form, consider working with a trainer or using mirrors to check your posture.

3. Start Light: Begin with lighter weights and gradually increase the resistance as you become more comfortable and stronger. It's better to start with less weight and focus on proper technique than to risk injury by lifting too heavy too soon.

4. Rest and Recovery: Give your muscles time to recover between workouts. Aim to strength train 2-3 times per week, allowing at least one day of rest between sessions for the same muscle group.

5. Listen to Your Body: Pay attention to how your body feels during and after exercise. It's normal to feel some muscle soreness, but sharp pain or discomfort could indicate an injury. If something doesn't feel right, stop and seek advice from a fitness professional or healthcare provider.

6. Stay Hydrated and Eat Well: Proper nutrition and hydration are essential for muscle recovery and overall performance. Make sure you're drinking enough water and eating a balanced diet rich in protein, healthy fats, and carbohydrates.

Creating a Strength Training Routine

1. Set Goals: Determine what you want to achieve with your strength training. Whether it's building muscle, increasing strength, or improving overall fitness, having clear goals can help you stay motivated.

2. Choose Exercises: Select a variety of exercises that target all major muscle groups, including legs, back, chest, shoulders, arms, and core. Aim for a balanced routine that works your entire body.

3. Plan Your Schedule: Decide how many days a week you can commit to strength training. A typical routine might include 2-3 sessions per week, with rest days in between.

4. Track Your Progress: Keep a workout journal to record the exercises you do, the weights you use, and how you feel. Tracking your progress can help you stay motivated and see how far you've come.

5. Mix It Up: Change your routine every few weeks to keep things interesting and to continue challenging your muscles. Try new exercises, increase the weights, or adjust the number of sets and reps.

Strength training is a powerful tool for building muscle, strengthening bones, and improving overall health. By understanding and using proper techniques, you can make your workouts more effective and safe. Whether you choose bodyweight exercises, free weights, weight machines, or resistance bands, incorporating strength training into your routine can help you achieve your fitness goals and enhance your quality of life.

Chapter 10: Weight-Bearing Exercises

Weight-bearing exercises are an excellent way to keep our bones strong and healthy. These exercises make you move against gravity while staying upright. They are especially important for preventing osteoporosis, a condition where bones become weak and brittle. Let's dive into why weight-bearing exercises are beneficial, explore different types of exercises, and learn how to incorporate them into your daily routine.

Why Weight-Bearing Exercises are Important

1. Build Bone Density: When you engage in weight-bearing activities, your bones and muscles work against gravity. This stress stimulates your bones to

build more cells, increasing their density and strength. Strong bones are less likely to break and can support your body better.

2. Prevent Bone Loss: As we age, our bones naturally lose density. Regular weight-bearing exercises help slow down this process, keeping our bones strong and reducing the risk of osteoporosis.

3. Improve Balance and Coordination: Many weight-bearing exercises also improve balance and coordination. This is crucial for preventing falls, which can lead to fractures, especially in older adults.

4. Boost Overall Health: These exercises also improve cardiovascular health, muscle strength, and flexibility. They can help with weight management, increase energy levels, and boost mood.

Types of Weight-Bearing Exercises

1. Walking and Hiking: Walking is one of the simplest and most effective weight-bearing exercises. It's easy to do and can be done almost anywhere. Hiking adds an extra challenge with varied terrain, which can increase bone and muscle strength.

2. Running and Jogging: These activities put more stress on your bones compared to walking, making them excellent for building bone density. Start with jogging and gradually increase to running as your fitness improves.

3. Dancing: Dancing is a fun way to strengthen your bones. It involves various movements that require your bones and muscles to work against gravity. Plus, it's a great way to enjoy music and socialize.

4. Stair Climbing: Whether you use a stair machine at the gym or take the stairs instead of the elevator, stair climbing is a powerful weight-bearing exercise. It targets the bones in your legs, hips, and spine.

5. Jumping Rope: This high-impact activity is great for building bone density, especially in your legs. It also improves coordination and cardiovascular fitness.

6. Team Sports: Sports like basketball, tennis, and soccer involve running, jumping, and quick changes in direction, all of which are weight-bearing activities. They are also a fun way to stay active and engage with others.

7. Weight Training: Lifting weights or using resistance bands can also be considered weight-bearing because they force your bones to work against an added weight. This can be done with free weights, weight machines, or resistance bands.

Incorporating Weight-Bearing Exercises into Your Routine

1. Start Slowly: If you're new to exercise or haven't been active for a while, start slowly. Begin with low-impact activities like walking and gradually progress to more challenging exercises like jogging or jumping rope.

2. Set Realistic Goals: Set achievable goals to keep yourself motivated. For example, aim to walk for 20 minutes three times a week and gradually increase the time and frequency.

3. Mix It Up: Incorporate a variety of weight-bearing exercises into your routine to work different parts of your body and keep things interesting. You might walk on some days, dance on others, and play a sport on the weekends.

4. Make It Social: Exercise with friends or join a group class. Having a workout buddy can make exercising more enjoyable and keep you accountable.

5. Stay Consistent: Aim for at least 30 minutes of weight-bearing exercise most days of the week. Consistency is key to building and maintaining bone density.

6. Listen to Your Body: Pay attention to how your body feels during and after exercise. It's normal to feel some muscle soreness, but sharp pain or discomfort could indicate an injury. If something doesn't feel right, stop and seek advice from a fitness professional or healthcare provider.

Tips for Safe and Effective Weight-Bearing Exercise

1. Wear Proper Footwear: Good shoes provide support and cushioning, which can help prevent

injuries. Make sure your shoes are appropriate for the activity you're doing.

2. Warm Up and Cool Down: Always start with a warm-up to prepare your muscles and joints for exercise. A few minutes of light cardio, like walking or marching in place, followed by dynamic stretches, can help prevent injuries. Cool down afterward with some gentle stretching to help your muscles recover.

3. Stay Hydrated: Drink plenty of water before, during, and after your workout. Staying hydrated is important for overall health and helps your body function properly during exercise.

4. Use Proper Form: Using the correct form is crucial to avoid injuries and get the most out of your workouts. If you're unsure about your form, consider working with a trainer or using mirrors to check your posture.

5. Listen to Your Body: Pay attention to how your body feels during and after exercise. It's normal to feel some muscle soreness, but sharp pain or discomfort could indicate an injury. If something doesn't feel right, stop and seek advice from a fitness professional or healthcare provider.

Making Exercise a Habit

1. Find Activities You Enjoy: Choose exercises that you like and look forward to. If you enjoy what you're doing, you're more likely to stick with it.

2. Schedule It In: Treat your exercise time like any other important appointment. Schedule it into your day and make it a priority.

3. Track Your Progress: Keep a workout journal to record your activities, how long you exercised, and how you felt. Tracking your progress can help you stay motivated and see how far you've come.

4. Celebrate Successes: Celebrate your achievements, no matter how small. Whether you walked an extra block or jogged for a few more minutes, recognizing your progress can boost your motivation.

5. Stay Positive: Focus on the positive aspects of exercise and how it makes you feel. Enjoy the journey and be kind to yourself.

Weight-bearing exercises are a vital part of maintaining strong and healthy bones. They help build bone density, prevent bone loss, and improve balance and coordination. By incorporating activities like walking, running, dancing, and weight training into your routine, you can enjoy the benefits of stronger bones and better overall health. Start slowly, set realistic goals, and find activities you enjoy to make weight-bearing exercise a regular part of your life. Stay consistent, listen to your body, and celebrate your successes along the way.

Chapter 11: Flexibility and Balance Training

Flexibility and balance training are essential components of a well-rounded fitness routine. They help improve your body's ability to move freely and maintain stability, which is important for daily activities and overall health. Let's explore why flexibility and balance are so important, look at different exercises, and learn how to incorporate them into your daily life.

Why Flexibility and Balance are Important

1. Improve Movement: Flexibility exercises stretch your muscles and improve the range of motion in your joints. This makes it easier to move and perform everyday tasks like bending down to tie

your shoes or reaching for something on a high shelf.

2. Prevent Injuries: Flexible muscles and joints are less likely to get injured. Stretching regularly can help prevent strains, sprains, and other injuries.

3. Enhance Performance: Whether you're playing sports, dancing, or just going for a walk, flexibility and balance can enhance your performance. They help you move more efficiently and with better coordination.

4. Reduce Pain: Regular stretching can help alleviate muscle tension and stiffness, reducing pain and discomfort, especially in areas like the lower back, neck, and shoulders.

5. Improve Posture: Flexibility exercises help lengthen tight muscles that can pull your body out of alignment. This can improve your posture and

reduce the risk of developing posture-related problems.

6. Boost Balance: Balance training strengthens the muscles that keep you stable, which is crucial for preventing falls. Good balance helps you stay steady on your feet and move with confidence.

Types of Flexibility Exercises

1. Static Stretching: This involves holding a stretch in a comfortable position for a period of time, usually 15-60 seconds. It's best to do static stretching after your muscles are warm, such as after a workout or a warm-up.

- Hamstring Stretch: Sit on the floor with one leg extended and the other bent. Reach toward your toes and hold the stretch. Repeat on the other side.
- Quadriceps Stretch: Stand on one leg, grab your opposite ankle, and pull it toward your buttocks. Hold the stretch and repeat on the other side.

- Shoulder Stretch: Bring one arm across your body and use your other arm to gently pull it closer. Hold the stretch and repeat with the other arm.

2. Dynamic Stretching: This involves moving parts of your body through a full range of motion in a controlled manner. It's great for warming up before physical activity.

- Leg Swings: Stand on one leg and swing the other leg forward and backward, then side to side. Repeat with the other leg.
- Arm Circles: Extend your arms to the sides and make small circles, gradually increasing the size. Reverse the direction after a few seconds.
- Torso Twists: Stand with your feet hip-width apart and twist your torso from side to side, letting your arms swing naturally.

3. Yoga: Yoga combines stretching with balance and relaxation techniques. It improves flexibility, balance, and mental focus.

- Downward Dog: Start on your hands and knees, then lift your hips toward the ceiling, forming an inverted V shape. Hold the position and breathe deeply.
- Child's Pose: Kneel on the floor, sit back on your heels, and stretch your arms forward, resting your forehead on the ground.
- Warrior Pose: Stand with your feet wide apart, turn one foot out, and bend the front knee. Extend your arms to the sides and hold the pose. Repeat on the other side.

4. Pilates: Pilates focuses on core strength, flexibility, and balance. It involves controlled movements and stretches.

- The Hundred: Lie on your back with your legs raised and your arms by your sides. Lift your head, neck, and shoulders off the ground and pulse your arms up and down while taking deep breaths.

- Spine Stretch Forward: Sit with your legs extended and your feet flexed. Reach forward toward your toes, rounding your spine, and then return to an upright position.

- Rolling Like a Ball: Sit with your knees bent and your feet off the ground, hugging your knees. Roll back onto your spine and then return to the starting position.

Types of Balance Exercises

1. Single-Leg Stands: Stand on one leg while lifting the other foot off the ground. Hold for 10-30 seconds and then switch legs. To make it more challenging, try closing your eyes or standing on a soft surface.

2. Heel-to-Toe Walk: Walk in a straight line, placing the heel of one foot directly in front of the toes of the other foot. This exercise improves your balance and coordination.

3. Balance Board or Stability Ball Exercises: Using a balance board or stability ball can add an extra challenge to your balance training. Try standing or sitting on the equipment while maintaining your balance.

4. Tai Chi: This ancient Chinese practice involves slow, controlled movements and deep breathing. Tai Chi improves balance, flexibility, and overall body control.

 - Basic Tai Chi Move: Stand with your feet shoulder-width apart and shift your weight to one foot. Slowly lift the opposite foot and step forward, then shift your weight to the other foot. Repeat with controlled movements.

Incorporating Flexibility and Balance Training into Your Routine

1. Stretch Daily: Make stretching a daily habit. Spend 5-10 minutes stretching your major muscle groups every day, either in the morning, before bed, or after your workout.

2. Practice Yoga or Pilates: Consider taking a yoga or Pilates class to improve your flexibility and balance. Many classes are available online, making it easy to practice at home.

3. Add Balance Exercises to Your Workouts: Include balance exercises in your regular workout routine. You can do them as part of your warm-up, during your strength training session, or as a standalone activity.

4. Be Mindful of Your Posture: Pay attention to your posture throughout the day. Stand and sit up

straight, engage your core muscles, and avoid slouching.

5. Stay Consistent: Consistency is key to seeing improvements in flexibility and balance. Aim to include these exercises in your routine at least a few times a week.

Tips for Safe and Effective Flexibility and Balance Training

1. Warm Up First: Always warm up before stretching to prevent injuries. A few minutes of light cardio, like walking or marching in place, can get your muscles ready for stretching.

2. Listen to Your Body: Stretch to the point of mild discomfort, not pain. If you feel sharp pain, ease off the stretch. Balance exercises should also be done carefully to avoid falls.

3. Use Props: If you're new to balance training, use props like a chair or wall for support until you feel more confident.

4. Wear Proper Footwear: Wear shoes that provide good support and grip, especially when doing balance exercises.

5. Progress Gradually: Start with basic exercises and gradually increase the difficulty as your flexibility and balance improve.

Making Flexibility and Balance Training a Habit

1. Set Goals: Set realistic and specific goals for your flexibility and balance training. For example, aim to touch your toes within a month or hold a single-leg stand for 30 seconds.

2. Track Your Progress: Keep a journal to record your exercises, how long you held each stretch, and

any improvements you notice. Tracking your progress can help you stay motivated.

3. Mix It Up: Incorporate a variety of exercises to keep things interesting. Try different stretches, balance drills, and activities like yoga or Tai Chi.

4. Stay Positive: Focus on the positive aspects of flexibility and balance training. Enjoy the feeling of stretching your muscles and the sense of accomplishment as your balance improves.

5. Reward Yourself: Celebrate your successes, no matter how small. Treat yourself to something you enjoy, like a relaxing bath or a favorite snack, after a good stretching session.

Flexibility and balance training are vital for maintaining a healthy, active lifestyle. They improve movement, prevent injuries, enhance performance, reduce pain, and boost overall well-being. By incorporating exercises like static and dynamic stretching, yoga, Pilates, and balance drills into your routine, you can enjoy the many benefits of improved flexibility and balance. Start slowly, set realistic goals, and stay consistent to make these exercises a regular part of your life.

Chapter 12: Developing a Personalized Exercise Plan

Creating a personalized exercise plan is one of the best things you can do for your health. A plan tailored to your needs, goals, and lifestyle can help you stay motivated, see results, and enjoy exercising. Let's explore how to develop an exercise plan that works for you, step by step.

Why a Personalized Exercise Plan is Important

1. Tailored to Your Goals: Whether you want to lose weight, build muscle, improve flexibility, or enhance your overall health, a personalized plan focuses on what you want to achieve.

2. Fits Your Lifestyle: A plan that fits your schedule and preferences is more likely to be sustainable. You can choose activities you enjoy and times that work best for you.

3. Keeps You Motivated: Knowing that your exercise plan is designed just for you can be highly motivating. It helps you stay committed and look forward to your workouts.

4. Tracks Progress: A personalized plan allows you to track your progress and make adjustments as needed. Seeing improvements can boost your confidence and encourage you to keep going.

Steps to Develop a Personalized Exercise Plan

1. Set Clear Goals

- Identify Your Objectives: What do you want to achieve? Do you want to lose weight, build strength, improve flexibility, or enhance your overall fitness? Be specific about your goals.

- Make Them Measurable: Set measurable goals so you can track your progress. For example, aim to lose 10 pounds, run a 5K, or do 20 push-ups in a row.

- Set a Timeline: Give yourself a realistic timeframe to achieve your goals. Having a deadline can keep you focused and motivated.

2. Assess Your Fitness Level

- Evaluate Your Current Fitness: Before starting, assess your current fitness level. You can do this through self-evaluation or with the help of a fitness professional.

- Know Your Limits: Understand your strengths and areas that need improvement. This will help you create a balanced plan that targets all aspects of fitness.

3. Choose Activities You Enjoy

- Find What You Like: Choose exercises and activities that you enjoy. Whether it's walking, running, swimming, dancing, or weightlifting, doing what you love makes it easier to stick with your plan.

- Mix It Up: Incorporate a variety of activities to keep things interesting. Mixing different types of exercise, like cardio, strength training, and flexibility exercises, ensures a well-rounded routine.

4. Create a Balanced Routine

- Include Different Types of Exercise: Aim for a balanced plan that includes cardiovascular exercise, strength training, flexibility exercises, and balance training.

- Cardio: Activities like walking, jogging, cycling, or swimming improve heart health and burn calories.

- Strength Training: Lifting weights, using resistance bands, or doing bodyweight exercises like push-ups and squats build muscle and strengthen bones.

- Flexibility: Stretching, yoga, or Pilates improve flexibility and reduce the risk of injuries.

- Balance: Balance exercises like standing on one leg or practicing Tai Chi improve stability and prevent falls.

5. Set a Schedule

- Plan Your Week: Decide how many days a week you will exercise and for how long. Aim for at least 150 minutes of moderate-intensity cardio each week, plus strength training on two or more days.

- Be Realistic: Choose a schedule that fits your lifestyle. If you're busy, short, more frequent workouts might be more manageable than longer sessions.

- Stay Consistent: Consistency is key. Try to stick to your schedule as closely as possible, but also be flexible if you need to adjust.

6. Start Slowly and Progress Gradually

- Ease Into It: If you're new to exercise or haven't been active for a while, start slowly. Gradually increase the intensity and duration of your workouts as your fitness improves.

- Listen to Your Body: Pay attention to how you feel during and after exercise. It's normal to feel some muscle soreness, but sharp pain or extreme fatigue may be a sign to slow down or adjust your plan.

7. Track Your Progress

- Keep a Journal: Record your workouts, including the type of exercise, duration, and how you felt. Tracking your progress helps you see improvements and stay motivated.

- Celebrate Milestones: Celebrate your achievements, no matter how small. Whether you ran an extra mile, lifted heavier weights, or simply felt more energetic, recognizing your progress can boost your confidence.

8. Make Adjustments as Needed

- Review Your Plan: Regularly review your exercise plan to see if it's working for you. If you're not seeing progress or your goals change, adjust your plan accordingly.

- Seek Professional Advice: If you're unsure about how to progress or make changes, consider consulting a fitness professional. They can provide guidance and help you optimize your plan.

9. Stay Motivated

- Find a Workout Buddy: Exercising with a friend can make workouts more enjoyable and keep you accountable.

- Join a Class or Group: Group classes or fitness communities can provide support, encouragement, and variety.

- Reward Yourself: Treat yourself to something you enjoy when you reach a goal. Whether it's a new workout outfit, a massage, or a favorite healthy snack, rewards can be a great motivator.

10. Enjoy the Journey

- Focus on the Positive: Enjoy the process of getting fit and healthy. Focus on how exercise makes you feel rather than just the end results.

- Stay Positive: Keep a positive attitude and be patient with yourself. Progress takes time, and every step forward is a victory.

Sample Exercise Plan

Here's a simple sample exercise plan to give you an idea of how to structure your routine:

Week 1-4

- Monday
  - 30 minutes of brisk walking
  - 10 minutes of stretching

- Tuesday

- 20 minutes of strength training (bodyweight exercises like push-ups, squats, and lunges)

- 10 minutes of balance exercises (standing on one leg, heel-to-toe walk)

- Wednesday
  - 30 minutes of cycling or swimming
  - 10 minutes of stretching

- Thursday
  - 20 minutes of strength training (using resistance bands or light weights)
  - 10 minutes of yoga or Pilates

- Friday
  - 30 minutes of dancing or another fun cardio activity
  - 10 minutes of stretching

- Saturday
  - 45 minutes of hiking or a long walk
  - 10 minutes of balance exercises

- Sunday

  - Rest day or gentle stretching/yoga

Week 5-8

- Monday

  - 40 minutes of jogging or running
  - 10 minutes of stretching

- Tuesday

  - 30 minutes of strength training (incorporating heavier weights or more challenging exercises)
  - 10 minutes of balance exercises

- Wednesday

  - 40 minutes of cycling or swimming
  - 10 minutes of stretching

- Thursday

  - 30 minutes of strength training (using resistance bands or light weights)

  - 15 minutes of yoga or Pilates

- Friday
  - 40 minutes of dancing or another fun cardio activity
  - 10 minutes of stretching

- Saturday
  - 1 hour of hiking or a long walk
  - 10 minutes of balance exercises

- Sunday
  - Rest day or gentle stretching/yoga

Developing a personalized exercise plan can transform your fitness journey. By setting clear goals, choosing activities you enjoy, and creating a balanced routine, you can make exercise a regular and enjoyable part of your life. Start slowly, track your progress, and make adjustments as needed. Stay motivated by celebrating your successes and focusing on the positive impact exercise has on your health and well-being. Remember, the journey to a healthier you is unique, and every step you take brings you closer to your goals.

Chapter 13: Lifestyle Changes for Bone and Muscle Health

Taking care of your bones and muscles is crucial for staying healthy and active as you age. Making a few simple changes in your lifestyle can have a big impact on your overall health. Let's explore some important lifestyle changes you can make to strengthen your bones and muscles, prevent osteoporosis, and improve your quality of life.

1. Eat a Balanced Diet

Eating a diet rich in nutrients is essential for bone and muscle health. Here are some key elements to focus on:

- Calcium: This mineral is vital for strong bones. Include calcium-rich foods like dairy products (milk, cheese, yogurt), leafy green vegetables (kale, broccoli), and fortified foods (orange juice, cereals) in your diet.

- Vitamin D: Vitamin D helps your body absorb calcium. You can get it from sunlight, fatty fish (salmon, mackerel), egg yolks, and fortified foods. Sometimes, a supplement might be necessary if you don't get enough from food and sunlight.

- Protein: Protein is important for muscle repair and growth. Include lean meats, poultry, fish, beans, lentils, nuts, seeds, and dairy products in your meals.

- Fruits and Vegetables: These are packed with vitamins, minerals, and antioxidants that support overall health, including bone and muscle health.

Aim to eat a variety of colorful fruits and vegetables every day.

- Whole Grains: Whole grains like brown rice, quinoa, and whole-wheat bread provide important nutrients and fiber. They help maintain a healthy weight, which is beneficial for your bones and muscles.

2. Stay Physically Active

Regular physical activity is crucial for maintaining strong bones and muscles. Here are some types of exercises to include in your routine:

- Weight-Bearing Exercises: Activities like walking, jogging, dancing, and hiking force you to work against gravity, which helps build bone strength.

- Strength Training: Lifting weights, using resistance bands, or doing bodyweight exercises like push-ups and squats help build muscle mass and strengthen bones.

- Flexibility Exercises: Stretching, yoga, or Pilates improve flexibility and reduce the risk of injuries. They also help maintain a good range of motion in your joints.

- Balance Exercises: Activities like Tai Chi, standing on one leg, or using a balance board improve stability and prevent falls, which is important for protecting your bones.

3. Avoid Smoking and Limit Alcohol

- Smoking: Smoking is bad for your bones and muscles. It reduces blood flow to the bones, weakens them, and increases the risk of fractures. Quitting smoking can significantly improve your bone health.

- Alcohol: Drinking too much alcohol can interfere with the body's ability to absorb calcium and can weaken your bones. Limit your alcohol intake to ensure your bones and muscles stay strong.

4. Maintain a Healthy Weight

- Weight Control: Keeping a healthy weight is important for your bones and muscles. Being underweight can increase the risk of fractures while being overweight puts extra stress on your bones and joints. Aim for a balanced diet and regular exercise to maintain a healthy weight.

5. Get Enough Sleep

- Rest and Recovery: Sleep is crucial for muscle recovery and overall health. Aim for 7-9 hours of quality sleep each night. Good sleep helps repair and rebuild muscles after exercise and supports overall well-being.

6. Manage Stress

- Stress Reduction: Chronic stress can negatively impact your bone and muscle health. Find ways to manage stress, such as practicing mindfulness, meditation, deep breathing exercises, or engaging in hobbies you enjoy.

7. Regular Health Check-ups

- Bone Density Tests: Regular check-ups with your doctor can help monitor your bone health. Bone density tests can detect osteoporosis early, allowing for timely treatment and prevention of further bone loss.

- Medication Review: Some medications can affect bone and muscle health. Discuss with your doctor any medications you're taking to understand their impact and explore alternatives if necessary.

8. Avoid Prolonged Sitting

- Move Often: Sitting for long periods can weaken your muscles and bones. Try to stand up, stretch, or walk around every hour, especially if you have a desk job.

9. Fall-Proof Your Home

- Safety Measures: To prevent falls, make your home safe. Remove tripping hazards, use non-slip mats, install grab bars in the bathroom, and ensure good lighting in all areas.

10. Wear Protective Gear

- Safety First: When engaging in activities that carry a risk of falling or injury, such as biking or certain sports, wear appropriate protective gear like helmets, knee pads, and elbow pads to protect your bones and muscles.

Putting It All Together

Making these lifestyle changes might seem overwhelming at first, but you can start with small steps and gradually build healthier habits. Here's how you can integrate these changes into your daily life:

- Start with One Change: Begin by focusing on one aspect, such as improving your diet or adding more physical activity to your routine. Once you're comfortable with that change, move on to the next.

- Set Realistic Goals: Set achievable goals for yourself. For example, aim to walk for 30 minutes a day, three times a week, and gradually increase the frequency and duration.

- Create a Routine: Establish a daily or weekly routine that includes healthy habits like exercise, balanced meals, and adequate sleep. Consistency is key to long-term success.

- Stay Positive: Focus on the benefits you're experiencing, such as increased energy, improved mood, or better sleep. Positive reinforcement can help keep you motivated.

- Seek Support: Share your goals with friends or family members who can provide support and encouragement. You might also consider joining a group or class for additional motivation.

Improving your bone and muscle health through lifestyle changes is a journey that requires commitment and consistency. By eating a balanced diet, staying active, avoiding harmful habits, and taking care of your overall well-being, you can build stronger bones and muscles and reduce the risk of osteoporosis. Remember, it's never too late to start making these changes. Every small step you take brings you closer to a healthier, stronger, and more active life. Stay focused, stay motivated, and enjoy the positive impact these changes will have on your health and quality of life.

Chapter 14: The Impact of Smoking and Alcohol

Smoking and drinking alcohol can have serious effects on your health, especially on your bones and muscles. Understanding these impacts can help you make better choices and improve your overall well-being. Let's explore how smoking and alcohol affect your body, particularly your bones and muscles, and why it's important to avoid or limit these habits.

How Smoking Affects Your Health

1. Weakens Bones: Smoking reduces blood flow to the bones, which can weaken them over time. This makes your bones more likely to break.

2. Interferes with Bone Growth: The chemicals in cigarettes can interfere with the body's ability to use calcium. Calcium is essential for building strong bones, and without enough of it, your bones can become brittle and fragile.

3. Slows Down Healing: Smoking slows down the healing process. If you break a bone or get injured, it will take longer to heal if you smoke.

4. Reduces Muscle Strength: Smoking can decrease the amount of oxygen that reaches your muscles. Muscles need oxygen to function properly, and without enough of it, they become weaker and tire more quickly.

5. Increases Risk of Osteoporosis: Osteoporosis is a condition where bones become weak and brittle. Smoking increases the risk of developing osteoporosis, especially in older adults.

6. Affects Overall Health: Besides impacting bones and muscles, smoking harms nearly every organ in the body. It increases the risk of heart disease, stroke, lung cancer, and many other serious health conditions.

How Alcohol Affects Your Health

1. Weakens Bones: Drinking too much alcohol can interfere with the body's ability to absorb calcium, which is vital for strong bones. This can lead to weaker bones and an increased risk of fractures.

2. Reduces Bone Density: Heavy drinking can reduce bone density, making bones more fragile and prone to breaking.

3. Impairs Muscle Growth: Alcohol can interfere with protein synthesis in muscles, which is essential for muscle growth and repair. This can lead to weaker muscles over time.

4. Dehydrates the Body: Alcohol dehydrates the body, and dehydration can affect muscle function. Muscles need adequate water to perform well, and without it, they can become cramped and weak.

5. Increases Risk of Falls: Drinking alcohol impairs coordination and balance, increasing the risk of falls and injuries. Falls can be particularly dangerous if your bones are already weakened.

6. Affects Overall Health: Excessive alcohol consumption can lead to liver disease, heart problems, and brain damage. It also weakens the immune system, making you more susceptible to infections.

Why It's Important to Avoid Smoking and Limit Alcohol

1. Better Bone Health: By avoiding smoking and limiting alcohol, you can help maintain stronger

bones. This reduces the risk of fractures and osteoporosis.

2. Stronger Muscles: Your muscles will be stronger and more efficient if they are not affected by the harmful effects of smoking and excessive drinking. This can improve your overall physical performance and reduce the risk of injuries.

3. Faster Healing: If you avoid smoking and limit alcohol, your body will heal more quickly from injuries. This is especially important as you age.

4. Improved Balance and Coordination: Limiting alcohol helps maintain better balance and coordination, reducing the risk of falls and related injuries.

5. Enhanced Overall Health: Avoiding smoking and limiting alcohol contribute to better overall health. This means a lower risk of chronic diseases

like heart disease, cancer, and liver disease, and a longer, healthier life.

Tips for Quitting Smoking and Limiting Alcohol

1. Set Clear Goals: Decide why you want to quit smoking or limit alcohol. Write down your reasons and refer to them when you need motivation.

2. Seek Support: Talk to friends, family, or a healthcare provider about your goals. They can provide encouragement and support.

3. Use Resources: There are many resources available to help you quit smoking and limit alcohol, including counseling, support groups, and medications.

4. Stay Busy: Find activities that keep you busy and distracted from the urge to smoke or drink.

Exercise, hobbies, and spending time with loved ones can be helpful.

5. Avoid Triggers: Identify situations that trigger your urge to smoke or drink and find ways to avoid or cope with them.

6. Reward Yourself: Celebrate your successes, no matter how small. Rewarding yourself can help you stay motivated and on track.

Smoking and drinking alcohol can have serious negative effects on your bones, muscles, and overall health. By understanding these impacts and making the choice to avoid smoking and limit alcohol, you can greatly improve your well-being. Your bones will be stronger, your muscles will function better, and your overall health will benefit.

Chapter 15: Stress Management and Its Effects

Stress is a common part of life. It can come from work, relationships, health problems, or even everyday challenges. While a little stress can be motivating, too much can harm your health, including your bones and muscles. Understanding how to manage stress effectively can improve your overall well-being. Let's explore what stress does to your body and how you can manage it to stay healthy.

How Stress Affects Your Body

1. Muscle Tension: When you're stressed, your muscles tense up. This is your body's way of protecting itself from injury. However, if you're

constantly stressed, your muscles remain tight, leading to pain and stiffness in areas like your neck, shoulders, and back.

2. Bone Health: Chronic stress can affect your bones. It can lead to the release of cortisol, a hormone that can weaken bones over time. High levels of cortisol can reduce bone density, increasing the risk of fractures and osteoporosis.

3. Immune System: Stress weakens your immune system, making you more susceptible to illnesses and infections. When your body is busy dealing with stress, it has less energy to fight off germs.

4. Sleep Problems: Stress can interfere with your sleep. Lack of sleep affects your body's ability to repair and build muscle and bone. Poor sleep can also make you feel tired and less motivated to exercise, which is important for maintaining bone and muscle health.

5. Digestive Issues: Stress can affect your digestive system, causing problems like stomach aches, constipation, or diarrhea. When your digestion is off, your body might not absorb the nutrients it needs to keep your bones and muscles strong.

6. Mental Health: Chronic stress can lead to anxiety and depression, which can affect your overall well-being. When you're mentally stressed, it's harder to stay active and make healthy choices for your bones and muscles.

Ways to Manage Stress

1. Exercise Regularly: Physical activity is one of the best ways to manage stress. Exercise releases endorphins, which are chemicals in the brain that act as natural painkillers and mood elevators. Activities like walking, jogging, yoga, and strength training can help reduce stress and improve your bone and muscle health.

2.   Practice Mindfulness and Meditation: Mindfulness involves focusing on the present moment without judgment. Meditation is a practice that helps calm the mind and reduce stress. Even a few minutes a day can make a big difference. Techniques include deep breathing exercises, guided imagery, or simply sitting quietly and focusing on your breath.

3. Get Enough Sleep: Aim for 7-9 hours of sleep each night. Good sleep helps your body repair and build muscle and bone. Establish a regular sleep routine, create a calming bedtime environment, and avoid screens before bed to improve your sleep quality.

4. Eat a Healthy Diet: Eating a balanced diet can help your body handle stress better. Include plenty of fruits, vegetables, whole grains, lean proteins,

and healthy fats in your meals. Avoid excessive caffeine and sugar, which can increase stress levels.

5. Stay Connected: Talking to friends and family can help you feel more supported and less stressed. Sharing your worries and getting a different perspective can make problems seem more manageable.

6. Take Breaks: Give yourself regular breaks during the day. Step away from your work or any stressful situation, even if it's just for a few minutes. Go for a walk, listen to music, or do something you enjoy to clear your mind.

7. Set Realistic Goals: Don't overload yourself with too many tasks. Break down big tasks into smaller, manageable steps. Prioritize what needs to be done and focus on one thing at a time.

8. Learn to Say No: It's okay to decline additional responsibilities if you're feeling overwhelmed. Saying no can help you manage your workload and reduce stress.

9. Stay Organized: Being organized can help you feel more in control and less stressed. Keep a calendar or to-do list to track your tasks and appointments.

10. Seek Professional Help: If stress feels overwhelming and you can't manage it on your own, seek help from a professional. A therapist or counselor can provide strategies to cope with stress and improve your mental health.

The Benefits of Managing Stress

1. Stronger Muscles and Bones: By managing stress, you reduce the levels of cortisol in your body, which helps maintain stronger bones and muscles. Regular exercise as a stress management technique

also directly benefits your muscle and bone strength.

2. Better Sleep: Stress management techniques can improve your sleep quality. Better sleep allows your body to repair and grow muscle tissue and bone.

3. Improved Immune Function: Reducing stress strengthens your immune system, making you less prone to illnesses that can weaken your body.

4. Enhanced Mental Health: Managing stress improves your mood, reduces anxiety, and can help prevent depression. A positive mental state makes it easier to stay active and make healthy choices.

5. Greater Energy Levels: Less stress means more energy. You'll feel more motivated to exercise and stay active, which is essential for maintaining healthy bones and muscles.

6. Better Digestion: When you manage stress effectively, your digestive system works better. This means your body can absorb more nutrients from food, which supports bone and muscle health.

Putting It All Together

Managing stress is not just about feeling better emotionally; it's also about taking care of your physical health. By incorporating stress management techniques into your daily routine, you can protect your bones and muscles and improve your overall well-being. Here are some steps to get started:

- Start Small: Begin with one or two stress management techniques that appeal to you. Gradually add more as you get comfortable with them.

- Be Consistent: Make stress management a regular part of your routine. Whether it's daily exercise, meditation, or setting aside time for relaxation, consistency is key.

- Listen to Your Body: Pay attention to how different techniques make you feel. Stick with the ones that work best for you and adapt as needed.

- Stay Positive: Remember that managing stress is a process. Celebrate your progress and be patient with yourself.

Managing stress effectively can have a profound impact on your bone and muscle health. By understanding how stress affects your body and implementing simple stress management techniques, you can strengthen your bones and muscles, improve your overall health, and enhance your quality of life.

Chapter 16: Monitoring Bone Density and Muscle Mass

Keeping track of your bone density and muscle mass is crucial for maintaining good health, especially as you age. Knowing how strong your bones and muscles are can help you take the right steps to prevent problems like osteoporosis and muscle loss. Let's explore why monitoring these aspects of your health is important, how to do it, and what the benefits are.

Why Monitoring is Important

1. Preventing Osteoporosis: Osteoporosis is a condition where bones become weak and brittle. By monitoring your bone density, you can catch early signs of bone loss and take steps to prevent it.

2. Maintaining Muscle Strength: Muscle mass naturally decreases with age, leading to weakness and increased risk of falls and injuries. Keeping an eye on your muscle mass can help you stay strong and active.

3. Detecting Changes Early: Regular monitoring helps you notice any changes in your bone density and muscle mass early on. Early detection allows for timely intervention, which can make a big difference in your health outcomes.

4. Guiding Your Exercise Routine: Knowing the state of your bones and muscles can help you tailor your exercise routine to your needs. For example, if your bone density is low, you might focus more on weight-bearing exercises.

5. Tracking Progress: If you're following a bone and muscle strengthening program, regular

monitoring can help you see the progress you're making. This can be motivating and encourage you to stick with your routine.

How to Monitor Bone Density

1. Bone Density Tests: The most common test for bone density is a DEXA scan (Dual-Energy X-ray Absorptiometry). This test is quick, painless, and provides accurate measurements of bone density. It's usually done at a medical facility and takes about 15 minutes.

2. Routine Check-ups: Regular check-ups with your doctor can include bone density assessments. Your doctor can recommend how often you should have these tests based on your age, gender, and risk factors.

3. Understanding Your Results: Bone density results are usually given as a T-score. A T-score of -1.0 or above is normal, between -1.0 and -2.5

indicates low bone density (osteopenia), and -2.5 or below suggests osteoporosis. Discuss your results with your doctor to understand what they mean for your health.

How to Monitor Muscle Mass

1. Body Composition Tests: These tests measure the amount of muscle, fat, and other tissues in your body. Methods include bioelectrical impedance analysis (BIA), skinfold measurements, and DEXA scans. BIA devices are often available at gyms or medical facilities and are quick and easy to use.

2. Strength Assessments: Simple strength tests, like measuring how many push-ups or squats you can do, can give you an idea of your muscle strength. These tests can be done at home and repeated regularly to track changes.

3. Physical Exams: During a physical exam, your doctor might assess muscle mass and strength

through simple tests like grip strength measurements or observing muscle tone and bulk.

4. Regular Exercise Monitoring: Keep track of your exercise routine and any changes in your physical capabilities. Noticing improvements in how much weight you can lift or how long you can exercise can indicate increases in muscle mass.

Benefits of Monitoring Bone Density and Muscle Mass

1. Personalized Health Plans: Monitoring helps create a personalized health plan that fits your needs. Whether it's adjusting your diet, increasing specific exercises, or taking supplements, you can make informed decisions based on your monitoring results.

2. Preventing Injuries: Strong bones and muscles reduce the risk of fractures and injuries. By

monitoring and maintaining your bone density and muscle mass, you can stay safer and more active.

3. Enhanced Quality of Life: Keeping track of these health metrics helps you stay independent and enjoy a higher quality of life. Strong bones and muscles make everyday activities easier and more enjoyable.

4. Motivation to Stay Active: Seeing positive changes in your bone density and muscle mass can be very motivating. It reinforces the benefits of your efforts and encourages you to keep going.

5. Better Aging: As you age, maintaining bone density and muscle mass becomes even more important. Regular monitoring helps you age gracefully, with fewer health problems related to weak bones and muscles.

Putting It All Together

1. Schedule Regular Tests: Talk to your doctor about scheduling regular bone density and muscle mass tests. Follow their recommendations on how often to have these tests based on your age and health status.

2. Keep a Health Journal: Write down your test results, exercise routines, and any changes you notice in your strength or mobility. This can help you track your progress and make adjustments as needed.

3. Stay Informed: Learn about the factors that affect bone density and muscle mass. Understanding how nutrition, exercise, and lifestyle choices impact your health can help you make better decisions.

4. Follow a Balanced Diet: Ensure your diet includes enough calcium, vitamin D, and protein, which are essential for bone and muscle health.

Consult a nutritionist if you need help planning a diet that supports your health goals.

5. Exercise Regularly: Incorporate weight-bearing exercises, strength training, and flexibility workouts into your routine. Aim for a balanced exercise plan that targets all major muscle groups and supports bone health.

6. Avoid Harmful Habits: Quit smoking and limit alcohol intake, as these can negatively affect bone density and muscle mass. Focus on healthy habits that support your overall well-being.

7. Seek Support: Join a fitness group or find a workout buddy to stay motivated. Having support can make it easier to stick to your exercise and health monitoring routine.

Monitoring your bone density and muscle mass is a proactive way to take charge of your health. By understanding the importance of these measures and regularly tracking them, you can make informed decisions that strengthen your bones and muscles, prevent health issues, and enhance your quality of life. Remember, it's never too late to start monitoring and improving your bone and muscle health.

Chapter 17: Working with Healthcare Providers

Your healthcare providers are important partners in maintaining your bone and muscle health. They have the knowledge and tools to help you understand your current health status, create a personalized plan, and monitor your progress. Working closely with them can make a significant difference in preventing and managing conditions like osteoporosis and muscle loss.

First, it's essential to communicate openly with your healthcare providers. Share your concerns and goals with them. Whether you're worried about your bone density, experiencing muscle weakness, or simply looking to improve your overall health, let them know. Your healthcare provider can offer valuable insights and recommend tests or treatments tailored to your needs.

Regular check-ups are a key part of this partnership. During these visits, your healthcare provider can assess your bone density and muscle mass through various tests. Bone density tests, such as DEXA scans, can detect early signs of bone loss. Muscle mass can be evaluated through body composition tests or simple strength assessments. These tests provide a baseline that helps track your progress over time.

In addition to tests, your healthcare provider can guide you in making lifestyle changes. They can recommend a balanced diet rich in essential nutrients like calcium, vitamin D, and protein. If necessary, they might suggest supplements to ensure you get the nutrients your bones and muscles need. They can also help you develop an exercise plan that includes weight-bearing exercises, strength training, and flexibility workouts, all crucial for maintaining strong bones and muscles. Your healthcare provider can also offer advice on managing other health conditions that might affect your bones and muscles. For example, if you have conditions like arthritis or diabetes, they can suggest strategies to minimize their impact on your bone and muscle health. They can also help you manage medications that might affect your bones and muscles, ensuring that you get the best possible outcomes from your treatment.

Don't hesitate to ask questions during your appointments. Understanding your health and the reasons behind your healthcare provider's recommendations can help you stay motivated and committed to your health plan. If something is unclear, ask for more information. Your healthcare provider is there to help you understand and make informed decisions about your health.

Building a good relationship with your healthcare provider is essential. Trust and open communication are the foundations of this relationship. Remember, your healthcare provider is on your side, working with you to achieve the best possible health outcomes. If you ever feel uncomfortable or unsure about their advice, seek a second opinion. It's important to feel confident in the care you're receiving.

Involving your healthcare provider in your health journey also means staying proactive. Follow their recommendations, attend regular check-ups, and keep them informed about any changes in your health. If you notice new symptoms or if something doesn't feel right, don't wait—contact your healthcare provider. Early intervention can prevent minor issues from becoming major problems.

Working with healthcare providers isn't just about treating existing conditions. It's also about prevention. By partnering with your healthcare provider, you can take steps to prevent bone and muscle problems before they start. Regular monitoring, a healthy lifestyle, and early intervention can keep your bones and muscles strong and healthy throughout your life.

Your healthcare providers are invaluable allies in your journey to maintain and improve your bone and muscle health. Through open communication, regular monitoring, and proactive care, you can work together to achieve your health goals.

Chapter 18: Preventing Falls and Fractures

Preventing falls and fractures is essential for maintaining your bone health, especially as you age. Falls can lead to serious injuries, including broken bones that can significantly impact your quality of life. By taking proactive steps to reduce the risk of falls, you can protect yourself and stay active and independent.

Understanding why falls happen is the first step in prevention. Many factors can increase your risk of falling. These include poor balance, weak muscles, vision problems, medications that cause dizziness, and hazards in your home. By addressing these factors, you can create a safer environment and reduce your risk.

Improving your balance is crucial. Activities like yoga and tai chi are excellent for enhancing balance and coordination. These exercises not only help you stay steady on your feet but also strengthen your muscles, which can prevent falls. Simple balance exercises, such as standing on one leg or walking heel-to-toe, can be done at home and incorporated into your daily routine.

Strength training is another important aspect of fall prevention. Strong muscles support your joints and help you maintain stability. Focus on exercises that strengthen your legs, core, and back. Squats, leg lifts, and core exercises like planks can make a big difference. Aim to include strength training in your routine at least two to three times a week.

Keeping your vision sharp is also vital. Regular eye exams can help detect vision problems early. If you need glasses, make sure your prescription is up-to-date and that you wear them as prescribed. Good lighting in your home, especially in stairways and hallways, can help you see better and avoid tripping over objects.

Reviewing your medications with your doctor can help identify any that might cause dizziness or balance issues. Some medications, especially those for high blood pressure, pain, or sleep, can increase your fall risk. Your doctor can adjust your medications or suggest alternatives to reduce this risk.

Creating a safe home environment is essential in preventing falls. Remove tripping hazards such as loose rugs, clutter, and electrical cords from walkways. Install grab bars in the bathroom, particularly near the toilet and in the shower or tub. Ensure that your home is well-lit, and consider using night lights in areas like the bathroom and bedroom.

Wearing appropriate footwear is another simple yet effective step. Choose shoes that fit well and provide good support. Avoid shoes with slippery soles or high heels, as these can increase your risk of falling. Non-slip socks can also be useful, especially if you prefer not to wear shoes indoors.

Staying active is key to maintaining your overall health and preventing falls. Regular physical activity keeps your muscles strong, improves your balance, and enhances your coordination. Activities like walking, swimming, and dancing are great options. Aim for at least 30 minutes of moderate activity most days of the week.

Listening to your body is important. If you feel unsteady or dizzy, take a moment to sit down and rest. Avoid rushing, especially when getting up from a chair or bed. Take your time to stand up slowly and steady yourself before walking. Using assistive devices like canes or walkers can provide extra support if you need it.

Educating yourself about fall prevention and staying informed about best practices can help you make better decisions. There are many resources available, including classes and workshops, that teach techniques for preventing falls and improving balance. Don't hesitate to seek out this information and apply it to your daily life.

Building a support network is also beneficial. Friends, family, and healthcare providers can offer assistance and encouragement. They can help you create a fall prevention plan and support you in staying active and safe. Don't be afraid to ask for help when you need it.

Preventing falls and fractures is an important part of maintaining your bone health and overall well-being. By improving your balance, strengthening your muscles, addressing vision and medication issues, creating a safe home environment, wearing appropriate footwear, staying active, and building a support network, you can significantly reduce your risk of falling. Taking these steps will help you stay independent, active, and healthy, allowing you to enjoy life to the fullest. Remember, fall prevention is an ongoing process, so keep making adjustments and improvements as needed. Your efforts will pay off in the form of stronger bones, better balance, and a higher quality of life.

Chapter 19: Special Considerations for Women

When it comes to bone and muscle health, women have unique challenges and needs. Understanding these differences can help women take proactive steps to maintain strong bones and muscles throughout their lives. From hormonal changes to lifestyle factors, several considerations can impact women's bone and muscle health.

One of the most significant factors affecting women's bone health is menopause. Menopause typically occurs in a woman's late 40s to early 50s, marking the end of her menstrual cycles. During menopause, the body's production of estrogen, a hormone that helps protect bones, decreases significantly. This drop in estrogen can lead to a rapid loss of bone density, increasing the risk of osteoporosis. Women can lose up to 20% of their bone density in the first five to seven years after menopause.

To counteract this, women should focus on building and maintaining bone density before and during menopause. A diet rich in calcium and vitamin D is crucial. Calcium is the building block of bones, while vitamin D helps the body absorb calcium. Foods like dairy products, leafy green vegetables, and fortified foods are excellent sources of calcium. Sun exposure and foods like fatty fish and fortified dairy products provide vitamin D.

Regular weight-bearing and resistance exercises are also essential. Activities like walking, jogging, dancing, and weightlifting can help maintain bone density and strengthen muscles. Incorporating these exercises into your routine can be particularly beneficial as you approach and go through menopause.

Hormone Replacement Therapy (HRT) is another option some women consider to manage menopausal symptoms and protect bone health. HRT involves taking estrogen or a combination of estrogen and progesterone to replace the hormones the body no longer produces. While HRT can help maintain bone density, it's not suitable for everyone and may carry risks. Discussing the benefits and risks with your healthcare provider is important to make an informed decision.

Pregnancy and breastfeeding are other life stages that can affect women's bone and muscle health. During pregnancy, a woman's body provides the developing baby with the necessary nutrients, including calcium. If a pregnant woman's diet lacks sufficient calcium, her body will take calcium from her bones to meet the baby's needs, potentially weakening her bones. Ensuring adequate calcium intake during pregnancy is vital for both the mother's and baby's health.

Breastfeeding also demands a higher intake of nutrients, including calcium and vitamin D. While breastfeeding, women should continue to focus on a nutrient-rich diet and consider supplements if recommended by their healthcare provider. Staying active with appropriate exercises can also help maintain muscle strength and support bone health during this period.

Another consideration for women is the impact of body weight on bone health. Being underweight can increase the risk of osteoporosis, as it may lead to lower bone density. Conversely, being overweight can put extra stress on bones and joints, potentially leading to other health issues. Maintaining a healthy weight through a balanced diet and regular exercise is crucial for bone and muscle health.

Certain lifestyle factors can also influence women's bone and muscle health. Smoking and excessive alcohol consumption can weaken bones and muscles. Smoking affects blood flow and nutrient delivery to the bones, while alcohol can interfere with the body's ability to absorb calcium. Quitting smoking and limiting alcohol intake can significantly improve bone and muscle health.

Women should also be mindful of their mental health. Chronic stress and anxiety can negatively impact physical health, including bone and muscle strength. Practicing stress management techniques, such as mindfulness, meditation, and regular physical activity, can help maintain overall well-being.

Regular check-ups with healthcare providers are essential for monitoring bone and muscle health. Women should discuss their risk factors for osteoporosis and other bone-related conditions with their doctors. Bone density tests, such as DEXA scans, can help detect early signs of bone loss and guide preventive measures.

For women with a family history of osteoporosis or other bone conditions, it's even more important to take proactive steps. Genetics can play a role in bone health, so being aware of family history and discussing it with your healthcare provider can help tailor a prevention plan that meets your needs.

Women face unique challenges in maintaining bone and muscle health, but with the right strategies, they can effectively manage these challenges. Understanding the impact of hormonal changes, focusing on a nutrient-rich diet, staying active, managing stress, and avoiding harmful habits are all crucial steps. Regular medical check-ups and open communication with healthcare providers can further support women in maintaining strong bones and muscles throughout their lives. By taking these proactive steps, women can protect their health and enjoy an active, fulfilling life.

Chapter 20: Bone and Muscle Health in Older Adults

As we age, maintaining bone and muscle health becomes increasingly important. For older adults, strong bones and muscles are key to staying active, independent, and healthy. However, the natural aging process can lead to a loss of bone density and muscle mass, making it essential to adopt strategies to combat these changes.

One of the most significant challenges older adults face is the natural decline in bone density. This decline can lead to osteoporosis, a condition where bones become weak and brittle, increasing the risk of fractures. Fractures in older adults can have serious consequences, often leading to reduced mobility and independence. Therefore, taking steps to maintain and improve bone health is crucial.

Calcium and vitamin D play a vital role in bone health. Calcium is a major component of bone tissue, and vitamin D helps the body absorb calcium. As people age, their ability to absorb calcium decreases, making it even more important to get enough of these nutrients. Older adults should aim to consume calcium-rich foods like dairy products, leafy greens, and fortified foods. Vitamin D can be obtained through sunlight exposure, but it's often necessary to take supplements, especially in regions with limited sunlight.

Regular exercise is another key factor in maintaining bone and muscle health. Weight-bearing exercises, such as walking, jogging, and dancing, help build and maintain bone density. Strength training exercises, such as lifting weights or using resistance bands, are crucial for maintaining muscle mass and strength. These exercises not only support bone health but also improve balance and coordination, reducing the risk of falls.

Falls are a major concern for older adults. A fall can lead to fractures, which can significantly impact an older person's quality of life. Preventing falls involves several strategies. First, improving balance through exercises like tai chi and yoga can help. These activities enhance coordination and stability, making falls less likely. Second, ensuring the home environment is safe is critical. Removing tripping hazards, installing grab bars in the bathroom, and using non-slip mats can make a big difference.

In addition to exercise and a safe home environment, maintaining a healthy diet is essential. Besides calcium and vitamin D, older adults need adequate protein to support muscle health. Protein is the building block of muscles, and getting enough protein can help prevent muscle loss. Lean meats, fish, beans, and nuts are excellent sources of protein. Incorporating a variety of these foods into the diet can help keep muscles strong.

Hydration is another important aspect of health that is often overlooked. Dehydration can lead to dizziness and weakness, increasing the risk of falls. Older adults should make a conscious effort to drink enough water throughout the day. Sometimes, the sense of thirst diminishes with age, so it's important to drink water regularly, even if not feeling thirsty.

Medications can also impact bone and muscle health. Some medications have side effects that affect balance, coordination, or bone density. It's important for older adults to review their medications regularly with their healthcare provider. Adjusting dosages or switching medications can sometimes reduce the risk of side effects that contribute to falls or bone loss.

Chronic conditions, such as arthritis and diabetes, can also affect bone and muscle health. Managing these conditions effectively is crucial. For example, arthritis can make it difficult to exercise, but low-impact activities like swimming can provide the benefits of exercise without putting too much strain on the joints. Managing blood sugar levels in diabetes is important to prevent complications that can affect the bones and muscles.

Mental health is another important consideration. Depression and anxiety can lead to decreased physical activity, which in turn can lead to weaker bones and muscles. Staying socially active, engaging in hobbies, and seeking help for mental health issues can improve overall well-being and support bone and muscle health.

Regular medical check-ups are essential for older adults. Bone density tests can help monitor bone health and detect early signs of osteoporosis. These tests provide valuable information that can guide treatment and prevention strategies. Healthcare providers can also recommend appropriate supplements and lifestyle changes to support bone and muscle health.

Maintaining bone and muscle health in older adults requires a comprehensive approach. A balanced diet rich in calcium, vitamin D, and protein, regular exercise, and a safe home environment are all crucial elements. Managing medications and chronic conditions, staying hydrated, and taking care of mental health are also important. Regular check-ups with healthcare providers ensure that any issues are detected and addressed early. By taking these steps, older adults can enjoy a higher quality of life, with strong bones and muscles that support an active and independent lifestyle. Remember, it's never too late to start taking care of your bone and muscle health. The efforts you make today can lead to a healthier and more fulfilling tomorrow.

Chapter 21: Managing Osteoporosis with Medication

Osteoporosis is a condition that weakens bones, making them fragile and more likely to break. While lifestyle changes such as diet and exercise are crucial for managing osteoporosis, medication can also play an important role. Understanding how these medications work and what they can do for you is essential for effectively managing this condition.

Several types of medications can help treat osteoporosis. These medications work in different ways to either slow bone loss or increase bone formation. Your doctor will help determine which medication is best for you based on your specific needs and health profile.

One common type of medication for osteoporosis is bisphosphonates. These drugs, which include alendronate (Fosamax), risedronate (Actonel), and zoledronic acid (Reclast), help prevent bone loss by slowing down the cells that break down bone. By reducing the activity of these cells, bisphosphonates help maintain or increase bone density. These medications are usually taken once a week, once a month, or even once a year, depending on the specific drug and its dosage.

Another type of medication is denosumab (Prolia). This drug is an injection given every six months and works by inhibiting the cells that break down bone. Denosumab can help increase bone density and reduce the risk of fractures in people with osteoporosis. It's particularly useful for individuals who cannot take bisphosphonates due to side effects or other health conditions.

Selective estrogen receptor modulators (SERMs), such as raloxifene (Evista), are another option. These medications mimic the positive effects of estrogen on bone density without some of the risks associated with estrogen therapy. SERMs can help maintain bone density and reduce the risk of spinal fractures.

For some people, hormone-related therapy might be an option. Hormone replacement therapy (HRT) can help maintain bone density by replacing estrogen in women who have gone through menopause. However, HRT carries some risks and is not suitable for everyone. It's important to discuss the benefits and risks with your doctor to determine if this treatment is right for you.

Another medication, teriparatide (Forteo), is a form of parathyroid hormone that stimulates new bone growth. Unlike other osteoporosis medications that mainly prevent bone loss, teriparatide helps build new bone. It is usually prescribed for people with severe osteoporosis or those who have not responded to other treatments. Teriparatide is given as a daily injection for up to two years.

Recently, another medication called romosozumab (Evenity) has been approved for osteoporosis treatment. This drug works by both increasing bone formation and decreasing bone breakdown. Romosozumab is given as a monthly injection for a year and has shown promising results in improving bone density and reducing fracture risk.

While these medications can be very effective, it's important to take them as prescribed and follow your doctor's instructions. Skipping doses or not taking the medication regularly can reduce its effectiveness and increase the risk of fractures. If you experience any side effects, such as stomach pain, difficulty swallowing, or muscle cramps, contact your doctor. They can help manage these side effects or adjust your treatment plan as needed.

In addition to medication, continuing with lifestyle changes is crucial for managing osteoporosis. A diet rich in calcium and vitamin D, regular weight-bearing and strength-training exercises, and avoiding smoking and excessive alcohol are all important parts of an osteoporosis management plan. These lifestyle changes complement the effects of medication and help keep your bones strong.

It's also important to have regular check-ups with your healthcare provider. Monitoring your bone density through tests like DEXA scans can help track your progress and determine if your treatment plan needs any adjustments. Your doctor may also check your blood levels of calcium and vitamin D to ensure you are getting enough of these nutrients.

Support from family and friends can also make a big difference. They can help remind you to take your medication, encourage you to stay active and support you in making healthy lifestyle choices. Joining a support group for people with osteoporosis can provide additional encouragement and share tips for managing the condition.

Remember, managing osteoporosis is a lifelong commitment. While medications can help significantly, they work best when combined with a healthy lifestyle and regular medical check-ups. Staying informed about your condition and working closely with your healthcare provider will help you make the best decisions for your bone health.

Managing osteoporosis with medication involves understanding the different types of drugs available and how they work. Bisphosphonates, denosumab, SERMs, hormone-related therapies, teriparatide, and romosozumab all offer various benefits in maintaining or improving bone density. Taking these medications as prescribed, alongside a healthy lifestyle and regular medical monitoring, can help you effectively manage osteoporosis and reduce the risk of fractures. Remember, you are not alone in this journey. With the right treatment and support, you can maintain strong bones and a good quality of life.

Chapter 22: Alternative Therapies and Treatments

While traditional medications and lifestyle changes are essential for managing bone and muscle health, some people explore alternative therapies and treatments. These alternatives can complement conventional treatments, offering additional ways to support your bone and muscle health. Understanding these options can help you make informed decisions about incorporating them into your overall health plan.

One popular alternative therapy is acupuncture. Acupuncture involves inserting thin needles into specific points on the body to stimulate healing and relieve pain. It has been used for thousands of years in traditional Chinese medicine. Some studies suggest that acupuncture can help manage pain associated with osteoporosis and arthritis, making it easier to stay active and maintain muscle strength. If you're interested in acupuncture, look for a licensed and experienced practitioner.

Another alternative treatment is chiropractic care. Chiropractors focus on the musculoskeletal system, especially the spine. They use hands-on spinal manipulation and other techniques to improve mobility and reduce pain. Chiropractic care can help alleviate back pain and improve posture, which is crucial for maintaining bone and muscle health. If you decide to try chiropractic care, ensure your chiropractor is licensed and has experience treating osteoporosis or other bone-related conditions.

Herbal supplements are also commonly used as alternative treatments. Some herbs, like black cohosh and red clover, are believed to have properties that can support bone health. These herbs may help balance hormones, particularly in women going through menopause, which can protect bone density. However, it's important to approach herbal supplements with caution. They can interact with medications and may not be suitable for everyone. Always consult your healthcare provider before starting any new supplement.

Another supplement gaining popularity is collagen. Collagen is a protein that helps build and maintain bones, muscles, skin, and tendons. Some research suggests that collagen supplements can improve bone density and joint health, making it easier to stay active and prevent falls. Collagen supplements are available in various forms, such as powders, pills, and liquids. When choosing a collagen supplement, look for high-quality products from reputable sources.

Essential oils are another alternative therapy some people use to support bone and muscle health. Oils like lavender, eucalyptus, and peppermint can be used in aromatherapy or applied topically (diluted with a carrier oil) to relieve pain and reduce inflammation. While essential oils cannot directly improve bone density, they can help manage symptoms like pain and stiffness, making it easier to maintain an active lifestyle.

Yoga and tai chi are alternative exercise practices that offer numerous benefits for bone and muscle health. Yoga involves a series of poses and stretches that improve flexibility, strength, and balance. Tai chi is a form of martial arts that involves slow, deliberate movements and deep breathing. Both practices help enhance balance and coordination, reducing the risk of falls. They also promote relaxation and stress reduction, which can positively affect overall health. Many community centers and fitness studios offer classes specifically designed for older adults or those with osteoporosis.

Massage therapy is another alternative treatment that can benefit bone and muscle health. Regular massages can help reduce muscle tension, improve circulation, and alleviate pain. This can make it easier to stay active and maintain muscle strength. When seeking massage therapy, choose a therapist experienced in working with individuals with osteoporosis or other bone conditions to ensure the techniques used are safe and effective.

Dietary changes and nutritional supplements are also essential components of alternative therapies. Some people explore specialized diets, like the anti-inflammatory diet, which focuses on reducing inflammation in the body through food choices. This diet includes plenty of fruits, vegetables, whole grains, and healthy fats while limiting processed foods and sugar. Reducing inflammation can help manage pain and improve overall health, supporting better bone and muscle function.

Mind-body practices, such as meditation and mindfulness, can also support bone and muscle health. Chronic stress can negatively impact your body, including your bones and muscles. Mindfulness and meditation techniques help reduce stress and promote relaxation. These practices can improve your mental well-being, making it easier to stick with healthy habits like regular exercise and proper nutrition.

It's important to remember that alternative therapies should not replace conventional treatments prescribed by your healthcare provider. Instead, they can be used in conjunction with traditional methods to enhance your overall health and well-being. Always communicate with your healthcare provider about any alternative therapies or supplements you are considering. They can help you understand the potential benefits and risks and ensure that these treatments are safe for your specific health condition.

Alternative therapies and treatments offer additional options for supporting bone and muscle health. Acupuncture, chiropractic care, herbal supplements, collagen, essential oils, yoga, tai chi, massage therapy, dietary changes, and mind-body practices can all play a role in maintaining strong bones and muscles. When used alongside

conventional treatments and lifestyle changes, these alternatives can enhance your
overall health and well-being.

Chapter 23: Success Stories and Case Studies

Real-life stories can inspire and motivate us to take action. Hearing how others have successfully managed their bone and muscle health can provide valuable insights and encouragement. In this chapter, we will share several success stories and case studies of individuals who have made significant improvements in their bone and muscle health. These stories highlight the importance of dedication, persistence, and the right strategies in achieving better health.

Mary's Journey to Stronger Bones

Mary, a 68-year-old retired teacher, was diagnosed with osteoporosis five years ago. Initially, she felt overwhelmed and worried about her future. Her doctor recommended a combination of medication, dietary changes, and exercise to manage her condition. Mary started taking bisphosphonate medication and incorporated more calcium and vitamin D-rich foods into her diet.

She also joined a local gym and began participating in weight-bearing and strength-training exercises three times a week. Mary found that she enjoyed group fitness classes, which kept her motivated and accountable. Over time, she noticed improvements in her strength and balance. Her regular bone density tests showed significant improvements, and her risk of fractures decreased.

Mary's dedication to her health and her willingness to follow her doctor's recommendations paid off. She now enjoys an active lifestyle, traveling and playing with her grandchildren without fear of fractures. Her story shows that with the right approach, it is possible to manage osteoporosis effectively and maintain a high quality of life.

John's Battle with Muscle Loss

John, a 72-year-old retired engineer, began experiencing muscle weakness and fatigue a few years ago. His doctor diagnosed him with sarcopenia, a condition characterized by the loss of muscle mass and strength due to aging. Determined to regain his strength, John started a comprehensive exercise program that included resistance training and aerobic activities.

John worked with a personal trainer who specialized in working with older adults. Together, they developed a personalized exercise plan that gradually increased in intensity. John also adjusted his diet to include more protein-rich foods, such as lean meats, fish, beans, and dairy products, to support muscle growth and repair.

After several months of consistent effort, John began to see remarkable improvements in his muscle strength and overall fitness. He could lift heavier weights, had better endurance, and felt more energetic throughout the day. John's success story illustrates the power of exercise and proper nutrition in combating muscle loss and improving overall health.

Susan's Holistic Approach to Osteoporosis

Susan, a 65-year-old yoga instructor, was diagnosed with osteoporosis despite her active lifestyle. She decided to take a holistic approach to managing her condition, combining conventional treatments with alternative therapies. Susan started taking medication prescribed by her doctor to slow bone loss and began incorporating more calcium and vitamin D into her diet.

In addition to conventional treatments, Susan explored alternative therapies such as acupuncture and herbal supplements. She also continued her regular yoga practice, focusing on poses that strengthen bones and improve balance. Susan's commitment to a holistic approach paid off. Her bone density improved, and she felt more balanced and grounded.

Susan's story highlights the importance of finding a personalized approach that works for you. By combining traditional and alternative treatments, she was able to manage her osteoporosis effectively and maintain her active lifestyle.

David's Transformation Through Lifestyle Changes

David, a 70-year-old former athlete, was shocked when he was diagnosed with osteoporosis. He had always been active and assumed his bones were strong. However, years of neglecting his diet and relying on high-impact sports had taken a toll on his bones. Determined to make a change, David overhauled his lifestyle.

He started by improving his diet, focusing on foods rich in calcium, vitamin D, and other essential nutrients. David also cut back on alcohol and quit smoking, both of which negatively impact bone health. He began a low-impact exercise routine that included swimming, cycling, and resistance training.

With the support of his family and healthcare team, David saw significant improvements in his bone density and overall health. He now serves as a mentor to others in his community, encouraging them to take proactive steps in maintaining their bone and muscle health. David's story demonstrates that it's never too late to make positive changes and improve your health.

Anna's Success with a Support Group

Anna, a 66-year-old librarian, struggled with staying motivated to manage her osteoporosis. She felt isolated and overwhelmed by her diagnosis. Her doctor suggested joining a support group for individuals with osteoporosis, and Anna decided to give it a try.

The support group became a crucial part of Anna's journey. She met others facing similar challenges, and they shared tips, recipes, and exercise routines. The group provided a sense of community and accountability that Anna had been missing. Encouraged by her peers, Anna started a regular exercise routine and improved her diet.

Over time, Anna's bone density stabilized, and she felt more confident in her ability to manage her condition. The support group not only helped her physically but also provided emotional support and encouragement. Anna's story highlights the power of community and the importance of seeking support when managing a chronic condition.

Tom's Experience with Medication and Lifestyle Changes

Tom, a 75-year-old retired professor, was diagnosed with osteoporosis after a fall that resulted in a fractured hip. Determined to prevent future fractures, Tom worked closely with his healthcare provider to develop a comprehensive treatment plan. He started taking medication to strengthen his bones and made significant changes to his diet and exercise routine.

Tom focused on weight-bearing exercises like walking and resistance training to build bone density and improve muscle strength. He also incorporated more calcium and vitamin D into his diet through dairy products, leafy greens, and supplements. Tom attended regular check-ups to monitor his progress and adjust his treatment plan as needed.

With persistence and dedication, Tom's bone density improved, and he regained his mobility and confidence. He now enjoys an active lifestyle, gardening, and playing with his grandchildren. Tom's story emphasizes the importance of combining medication with lifestyle changes to effectively manage osteoporosis and improve overall health.

These success stories and case studies show that managing bone and muscle health is possible with the right strategies and support. Whether through medication, lifestyle changes, alternative therapies, or community support, individuals can take proactive steps to improve their bone and muscle health and lead fulfilling lives.

Conclusion

Taking care of your bones and muscles is essential for leading a healthy, active, and fulfilling life. This book has provided a comprehensive guide to understanding the importance of bone and muscle health, the science behind it, and the various strategies you can use to strengthen them. From nutrition and exercise to alternative therapies and medication, there are many ways to support your bone and muscle health.

As we've seen in the success stories and case studies, managing conditions like osteoporosis is achievable with the right approach and commitment. It's about creating a personalized plan that works for you, staying consistent with your efforts, and seeking support when needed. Whether you're just starting to think about your bone and muscle health or have been managing a condition for years, it's never too late to make positive changes.

Remember, small steps can lead to big improvements. Incorporating calcium and vitamin D into your diet, engaging in regular physical activity, and making lifestyle changes such as quitting smoking and reducing alcohol consumption can all have a significant impact on your bone and muscle health. Additionally, exploring alternative therapies and staying informed about new treatments can provide additional benefits.

Your healthcare provider is a valuable partner in this journey. Regular check-ups, bone density tests, and open communication with your doctor will help you stay on track and make any necessary adjustments to your plan. Don't hesitate to ask questions and seek guidance as you work towards your health goals.

Maintaining strong bones and muscles is a lifelong commitment that requires dedication, knowledge, and support. By following the advice and strategies outlined in this book, you can take control of your bone and muscle health and enjoy a higher quality of life. Embrace the journey, stay positive, and remember that every step you take brings you closer to a healthier, more active you. Your bones and muscles will thank you for the care and attention you give them, allowing you to live life to the fullest.